HUMANIZING BRAIN TUMORS

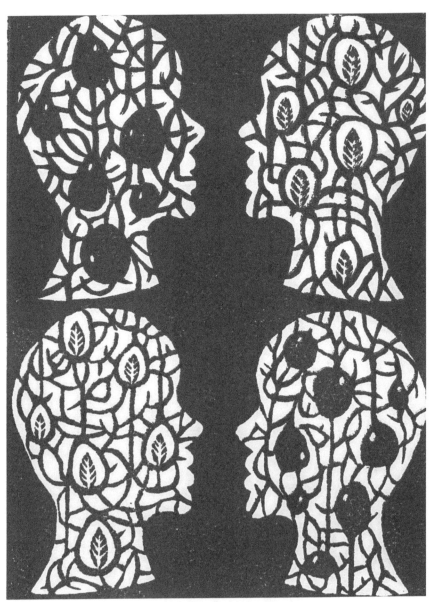

by Shivani Ghoshal, MD

HUMANIZING BRAIN TUMORS

Strategies for You and Your Physician

EDITED BY

JONATHAN A. FORBES, MD

ABDELKADER MAHAMMEDI, MD

SOMA SENGUPTA, MD, PHD, FRCP

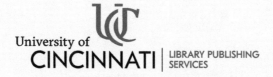

University of
CINCINNATI | LIBRARY PUBLISHING
SERVICES

About the University of Cincinnati Library Publishing Services (CLIPS)
CLIPS provides professional publishing services for digital and print publications, conference proceedings, journals, affordable textbooks and open educational resources produced by University of Cincinnati faculty, staff and organizations with department sponsorship and funding. CLIPS encourages authors to publish in barrier-free open access formats. CLIPS in an imprint of the University of Cincinnati Press, which is committed to publishing rigorous, peer-reviewed, leading scholarship in social justice, community engagement, and Cincinnati/Ohio history.

University of Cincinnati Press
Copyright © 2022
An enhanced open-access edition of this book is available at:
https://ucincinnatipress.manifoldapp.org/projects/humanizing-brain-tumors

Requests regarding this work should be sent to University of Cincinnati Press, Langsam Library, 2911 Woodside Drive, Cincinnati, Ohio 45221
ucincinnatipress.uc.edu

ISBN 978-1-947603-60-8 (paperback)
ISBN 978-1-947603-61-5 (open access)
ISBN 978-1-947603-59-2 (e-book, EPUB)
DOI: 10.34314/humanizingbrain.00001

LCCN: 2021952548

Designed and produced for UC Press by Julie Rushing
Typeset in Scala Sans Pro and Scala Pro
Printed in the United States of America
First Printing

Front cover image (detail) and frontispiece by Shivani Ghoshal, MD

This book is dedicated to brain tumor patients and their families. Each patient has a special journey that makes their story unique and educational for readers.

CONTENTS

PREFACE

SOMA SENGUPTA, MD, PHD, FRCP

n 1884, Rickman Godlee surgically removed a glioma from a patient in London, England. Although it was an important moment in the history of medicine, the patient unfortunately died twenty-eight days after surgery due to meningitis and other complications. Neurosurgery has come a long way from the times of Rickman Godlee. Without question, then as much as now, the true heroes are the courageous patients with brain tumors and their critical support network of family and friends. Dr. Forbes, Dr. Mahammedi, and I sincerely hope this book will serve as both an educational reference and a source of inspiration for brain tumor patients and their families. We are clinician-researchers who share the scientific and medical community's relentless pursuit of perfecting treatment for every type of brain tumor. Dr. Forbes has had a family member affected by a brain tumor, and I have had family members and a close friend affected by brain tumors as well.

With the COVID-19 pandemic causing lockdowns, 2020 and 2021 were unusual years that changed the way we educated students. We felt the need to create a project for medical students who could no longer rotate in science laboratories or clinical settings but still yearned to learn. What better way to learn than writing and thinking about patient journeys? We also felt the need to tell the real stories of our patients, who felt that their symptoms were initially ignored before they were diagnosed with brain tumors. Often, family and emergency room physicians, and medical residents, fellows, and students are not aware of the different presentations brain tumors may have in patients have. In addition, brain tumor patients need a place where they can feel "not alone"—where others have been through similar experiences. Patients with a new brain tumor diagnosis may also want to find a place of connection with resources they can consult. We hope this book will serve as that place.

To this end, we wrote a book with nine case studies, and we had a diverse team contribute, including physicians, medical students, and residents. It is important that the next generation of physicians is exposed to the journeys of patients. If they cannot be at the bedside, they can learn through the trials and tribulations of each patient. This was a highly interactive book where we interviewed the patients and or their families to piece together the story from the perspective of the patient and their family members.

When I discussed this project with my collaborator and friend, Jonathan Forbes, we never imagined that we would actually be where we are today. As a neuro-oncologist, I wanted to be more than a person who recommended chemotherapy and clinical trials, while Jonathan Forbes, a neurosurgeon, wanted to be more than a person who resected brain tumors. We both wanted to understand our patients, do translational research, and educate students as the next generation of scientists and physicians. We decided to produce this open access book from the generosity of patients and their families, in particular, Columbus (Chapter 2), Jan (Chapter 3), and Beth's (Chapter 5) families.

Columbus, Jan, and Beth were my patients. Each wanted their experiences shared and their stories told. In the pages that follow, you will meet Columbus, the brave veteran who became an artist. He traveled from Atlanta with his wife, Val, and their daughters to join in the Walk Ahead for a Brain Tumor Cure walk in 2019, a major annual event that raises funds for the University of Cincinnati Gardner Neuroscience Institute Brain Tumor Center. You will meet Jan, the child who loved watching NASA rocket launches at Cape Canaveral, who liked lobster fishing, traveling, playing musical instruments, and who so bravely battled cancer twice. And beautiful Beth, the dedicated bone marrow transplant nurse, whose life was snuffed out like a candle's fickle flame. All of these wonderful patients, and many others, never cease to inspire.

Dr. Oliver Sacks, a British neurologist who died of cancer in 2015, once said: "I feel intensely alive, and I want and hope in the time that remains to deepen my friendships, to say farewell to those I love, to write more, to travel if I have the strength, to achieve new levels of understanding and insight." This is what many of our inspiring patients have told us. So, we dedicate this book to patients, their families, and their journeys. We, as physicians, journey with them. As the former U.S. Senator Ted Kennedy, who died of a glioblastoma, once said, "For all those whose cares have been our concern, the work goes on, the cause endures, the hope still lives, and the dream shall never die."

HUMANIZING BRAIN TUMORS

CHAPTER 1

FRONTAL LOBE
The Man Who Lost the Will to Work

ZOE ANDERSON, MS

CHITRA KUMAR, BA

MARK JOHNSON, MD

JONATHAN A. FORBES, MD

The human frontal lobe comprises approximately 35-40% of the volume of the cerebral hemispheres.[1] It is thus perhaps not surprising that this region of the brain subserves many critical functions. On the dominant side, the inferior part of the frontal lobe (known as Broca's area, a region of the inferior frontal gyrus) is the center of speech and language production.[2] A region of the posterior frontal lobe known as primary motor cortex controls motor function on the opposite side of the body. Other portions of the frontal lobe, including the prefrontal cortex, promote empathy, attention to detail, and motivation and form the basis for decision making, personality, and problem-solving capacity.[3] Depending on the specific region involved, damage to the frontal lobe can manifest in many different ways. As an example, damage to the posterior right frontal lobe (primary motor cortex) can result in severe left sided weakness. Significant damage to prefrontal cortex can cause a person to become more impulsive or not function appropriately in social situations.[4] One famous example of the relationship between frontal lobe structure and function is the story of Phineas Gage, an American foreman whose left frontal lobe was impaled by a tamping iron following a railroad blast injury in 1848.[5] The iron was able to be successfully removed. Incredibly, Gage was able to recover from the injury.

Following his convalescence, many observers noted marked changes in Gage's personality.[6] Specifically, Gage was reported to have become impulsive and uninhibited—now unable to keep a job. This famous anecdote is a reminder of the complex relationship that exists between frontal lobe function and personality/executive behavior. Changes like those noted in Phineas Gage are often observed by friends and family members of patients who have suffered severe damage to the frontal lobe(s).[7]

In the case of Phineas Gage, penetrating injury from a tamping rod resulted in frontal lobe injury. It is important to remember that, infrequently, damage to the frontal lobe can develop in individuals with no history of trauma—occasionally from unexpected causes like brain tumors. Meningiomas, which arise from the leathery covering of the brain and spinal cord, are an important type of brain tumor that can result in progressive and insidious injury to the frontal lobes. Meningiomas are the most common *primary* brain tumor—accounting for roughly 35% of primary brain tumors diagnosed each year.[8] Approximately 10% of intracranial meningiomas arise from a region of the skull base known as the olfactory groove.[9] While the vast majority of olfactory-groove meningiomas (OGM) are benign and slow-growing, these tumors can sometimes become very large after many years of undetected growth. As frontal lobe dysfunction associated with large OGMs often results in somewhat vague and non-specific symptoms, it is not uncommon for patients to go very long periods of time before these tumors are identified. When massive, OGMs sometimes progress to compress the optic apparatus posteroinferiorly—symptoms that often lead to imaging and prompt detection.[10] In the following paragraphs, you will hear more about Robert*: one such patient whose personality, independence, ability to hold a job, and executive function deteriorated over the course of many years. Ultimately, when Robert's vision started to decline, an MRI ordered by his treating physician identified a massive OGM found to be compressing and damaging both frontal lobes.

----

* a pseudonym

In his 40s, Robert was a successful actor in the Cincinnati community, having starred in many successful musicals. At the peak of his career, his friends and family members described him as energetic, meticulous, and a dynamic performer. As he aged, many around him noted that Robert seemed to care progressively less about specific details. Robert's performance as an actor began to gradually decline. Eventually, friends and family were forced to place Robert in an assisted-living facility, under the supervision of a caregiver. Because he suffered from type II diabetes, Robert required an annual visit to his eye doctor or ophthalmologist. On one such visit, Robert's vision, which previously had been perfect, was noted to have gotten slightly worse. New, minor visual loss involving the temporal field of the left eye was detected. Robert's ophthalmologist initially felt that he might be suffering from glaucoma, a common eye condition caused by increased pressure in the eye. However, additional testing was negative for increased intraocular pressure. As the visual loss was minimal, and Robert didn't seem to be particularly concerned, the medical team decided to monitor conservatively. Over the next few years, the vision in Robert's left eye deteriorated further, and he began to lose vision in the temporal field of his right eye as well. Formal testing demonstrated that Robert's now had bitemporal hemianopsia, a pattern of visual loss in the outer half of the visual fields in both eyes known to be concerning for a structural or compressive etiology.

During the same period of time his vision had inexplicably worsened, Robert's caregiver began to notice additional changes in his personality. Every day, Robert seemed a little less like himself. He was sleeping more than usual and now missing many of the community events he would previously attend. When Robert stopped checking his blood sugar levels and taking his medications, his caregiver felt something was very wrong. In light of both the vision and personality changes, Robert was ultimately referred to a neurologist. In addition to Robert's deterioration in vision and personality, detailed neurologic testing in neurologic clinic also revealed anosmia or loss of smell with associated deterioration in taste. Anosmia is yet another symptom commonly observed with massive OGMs that often goes initially undetected; progressive enlargement of olfactory groove meningiomas stretches the olfactory nerve(s), often resulting in loss of smell in large or massive OGMs.[11] Following thorough evaluation in neurology clinic, magnetic resonance imaging (MRI) of the brain was ordered. These images demonstrated a massive tumor originating from the olfactory groove (Figure 1.1). The tumor extended posteriorly to compress Robert's optic chiasm—explaining his progressive visual loss. The massive tumor could also be seen to displace and compress both frontal lobes, providing an explanation for the pronounced changes in personality and executive function his family and caregivers had noted. On MRI, the appearance of the tumor was most consistent with an olfactory groove meningioma.

After the report from the MRI returned, Robert was referred to Dr. Jonathan Forbes, a neurosurgeon specializing in skull base tumors. Dr. Forbes explained to Robert that, without surgery, the tumor would continue to grow and further impair his vision and personality. With surgery, Robert's vision was likely to improve. It was also likely that removal of the tumor would help Robert regain some element of frontal lobe function. Though hearing about the surgery was scary, Robert and his family knew the tumor had to be removed (Figure 1.1A). Dr. Forbes performed a technique often used for large tumors in the anterior skull base called a bifrontal craniotomy (Figure 1.1B).[12] After removing a portion of the skull

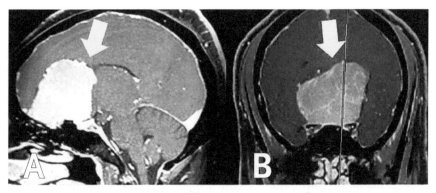

FIGURE 1.1   MRI demonstrating Robert's olfactory groove meningioma. Sagittal (A) and coronal (B) images demonstrate a massive olfactory groove meningioma (yellow arrow) resulting in severe compression of the frontal lobe and vital optic structures required for vision.

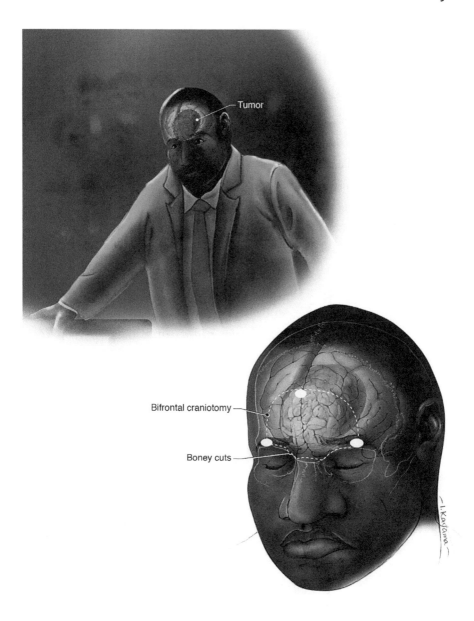

FIGURE 1.2 Robert suffered many unusual personality changes as he aged. His performance as an actor began to decline and eventually he required placement in an assisted-living facility. A surgery known as an extended bifrontal craniotomy was used to remove the tumor. The boney cuts necessary for tumor removal can be visualized in this figure.

bone covering the frontal lobes, he opened the dura mater—the tough outermost layer of the meninges covering the brain. The tumor was de-vascularized from its origin along the olfactory groove and debulked using a device called a sonopet. The tumor could then be meticulously dissected from adjacent healthy brain tissue. With the aid of high magnification, Dr. Forbes carefully dissected the tumor from Robert's optic nerves and pituitary stalk. The entire tumor was removed and sent to pathology, confirming a benign meningioma.

Robert did well after the surgery, noting instantaneous improvement in vision, and was discharged after a few days in the hospital. A year after his surgery, Robert returned for a follow-up appointment. Repeat MRI showed no trace of any residual or recurrent tumor (Figure 1.3). At this time, both Robert and his caregiver had noted considerable improvement in Robert's personality and level of executive function. One year following surgery, Robert felt more like himself again. He had regained the capacity to cook his meals and check his blood sugar daily. For Robert, however, the best part of his recovery was finding a way to return to help with the community plays he loved so much.

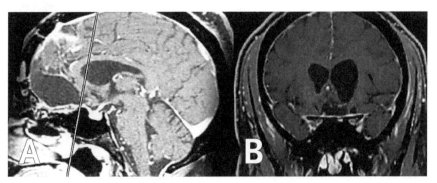

FIGURE 1.2 MRI obtained one year following surgery. Post-operative sagittal (A) and coronal (B) MR images continue to demonstrate no evidence of residual or recurrent tumor.

ENDNOTES

1. Celine Chayer and Morris Freedman, "Frontal Lobe Functions," *Current Neurology and Neuroscience Reports* 1, no. 6 (November 2001): 547. https://doi.org/10.1007/s11910-001-0060-4.

2. Paul Broca, "Nouvelle observation aphémie produite par un lésion de la moité postérieure des deuxiéme et troisiéme circonvolutions frontales," *Bullentins de la Socie'te' Anatomique* 6, (1861): 398-40; Paul Broca, "Localisation des fonctions cérébrales. Siége du langage articulé." *Bulletins de la Société d' Anthropologie* 4, (1863): 200-204.

3. María Roca et al., "Executive Function and Fluid Intelligence after Frontal Lobe Lesions," *Brain: A Journal of Neurology* 133, no. 1 (January 2010): 234–47. https://doi.org/10.1093/brain/awp269.

4. Raghavan Sheelakumari et al., "Neuroanatomical correlates of apathy and disinhibition in behavioural variant frontotemporal dementia," *Brain Imaging Behavior* 14, no. 5 (2020): 2004-2011. https://doi.org/10.1007/s11682-019-00150-3.

5. John M. Harlow, "Passage of an iron rod through the head," *Boston Medical and Surgical Journal* 39, (1848): 389-393.

6. Harlow, "Passage of an iron rod through the head," 389-393.

7. John M. Harlow, "Recovery from the passage of an iron bar through the head," *Publications of the Massachusetts Medical Society* 2, (1868): 327-347.

8. Christine Marosi et al., "Meningioma," *Critical Reviews in Oncology/Hematology* 67, no. 2 (August 1, 2008): 153–71. https://doi.org/10.1016/j.critrevonc.2008.01.010; Joseph Wiemels, Margaret Wrensch, and Elizabeth B. Claus, "Epidemiology and Etiology of Meningioma," *Journal of Neuro-Oncology* 99, no. 3 (September 2010): 307–14. https://doi.org/10.1007/s11060-010-0386-3.

9. Stephen J. Hentschel and Franco DeMonte, "Olfactory Groove Meningiomas," *Neurosurgical Focus* 14, no. 6 (June 1, 2003): 1–5. https://doi.org/10.3171/foc.2003.14.6.4.

10. Alexandru Vlad Ciurea et al., "Olfactory Groove Meningiomas," *Neurosurgical Review* 35, no. 2 (April 1, 2012): 195–202. https://doi.org/10.1007/s10143-011-0353-2; A. Tsikoudas and D. P. Martin-Hirsch, "Olfactory Groove Meningiomas," *Clinical Otolaryngology & Allied Sciences* 24, no. 6 (1999): 507–9. https://doi.org/10.1046/j.1365-2273.1999.00303.x.

11. A. Welge-Luessen, "Olfactory Function in Patients with Olfactory Groove Meningioma," *Journal of Neurology, Neurosurgery & Psychiatry* 70, no. 2 (February 1, 2001): 218–21. https://doi.org/10.1136/jnnp.70.2.218.

12. Makoto Nakamura et al., "Olfactory Groove Meningiomas: Clinical Outcome and Recurrence Rates after Tumor Removal through the Frontolateral and Bifrontal Approach," *Neurosurgery* 60, no. 5 (May 2007): 844–52.

REFERENCES

Broca, Paul. "Nouvelle observation aphémie produite par un lésion de la moité postérieure des deuxiéme et troisiéme circonvolutions frontales." *Bullentins de la Socie'te' Anatomique* 6, (1861): 398-407

Broca, Paul. "Localisation des fonctions cérébrales. Siége du langage articulé." *Bulletins de la Sociétéd' Anthropologie* 4, (1863): 200-204

Chayer, Celine, and Morris Freedman. "Frontal Lobe Functions." *Current Neurology and Neuroscience Reports* 1, no. 6 (November 2001): 547–52. https://doi.org/10.1007 /s11910-001-0060-4.

Ciurea, Alexandru Vlad, Stefan Mircea Iencean, Radu Eugen Rizea, and Felix Mircea Brehar. "Olfactory Groove Meningiomas." *Neurosurgical Review* 35, no. 2 (April 1, 2012): 195–202. https://doi.org/10.1007/s10143-011-0353-2.

Harlow, John M. "Passage of an iron rod through the head." *Boston Medical and Surgical Journal* 39, (1848): 389-393.

Harlow, John M. "Recovery from the passage of an iron bar through the head." *Publications of the Massachusetts Medical Society* 2, (1868): 327-347.

Hentschel, Stephen J., and Franco DeMonte. "Olfactory Groove Meningiomas." *Neurosurgical Focus* 14, no. 6 (June 1, 2003): 1–5. https://doi.org/10.3171/foc.2003.14.6.4.

Marosi, Christine, Marco Hassler, Karl Roessler, Michele Reni, Milena Sant, Elena Mazza, and Charles Vecht. "Meningioma." *Critical Reviews in Oncology/Hematology* 67, no. 2 (August 1, 2008): 153–71. https://doi.org/10.1016/j .critrevonc.2008.01.010.

Nakamura, Makoto, Melena Struck, Florian Roser, Peter Vorkapic, and Madjid Samii. "Olfactory Groove Meningiomas: Clinical Outcome and Recurrence Rates after Tumor Removal through the Frontolateral and Bifrontal Approach." *Neurosurgery* 60, no. 5 (May 2007): 844–52; discussion 844-852. https://doi.org/10.1227/01.NEU .0000255453.20602.80.

Roca, María, Alice Parr, Russell Thompson, Alexandra Woolgar, Teresa Torralva, Nagui Antoun, Facundo Manes, and John Duncan. "Executive Function and Fluid Intelligence after Frontal Lobe Lesions." *Brain: A Journal of Neurology* 133, no. 1 (January 2010): 234–47. https://doi.org/10.1093/brain/awp269.

Sheelakumari, Raghavan, Cheminnikara Bineesh, Tinu Varghese, Chandrasekharan Kesavadas, Joe Verghese, and Pavagada S. Mathuranath. "Neuroanatomical correlates of apathy and disinhibition in behavioural variant frontotemporal dementia." *Brain Imaging Behavior* 14, no. 5 (2020): 2004-2011. https://doi.org/10.1007 /s11682-019-00150-3.

Tsikoudas, A., and D. P. Martin-Hirsch. "Olfactory Groove Meningiomas." *Clinical Otolaryngology & Allied Sciences* 24, no. 6 (1999): 507–9. https://doi .org/10.1046/j.1365-2273.1999.00303.x.

Welge-Luessen, A. "Olfactory Function in Patients with Olfactory Groove Meningioma." *Journal of Neurology, Neurosurgery & Psychiatry* 70, no. 2 (February 1, 2001): 218–21. https://doi.org/10.1136/jnnp.70.2.218.

Wiemels, Joseph, Margaret Wrensch, and Elizabeth B. Claus. "Epidemiology and Etiology of Meningioma." *Journal of Neuro-Oncology* 99, no. 3 (September 2010): 307–14. https://doi.org/10.1007/s11060-010-0386-3.

CHAPTER 2

LEFT TEMPORAL LOBE
The Man Who Found Creativity

ABIGAIL KOEHLER, BS

ROHAN RAO, BS

YANA TOMASSIAN

ABDELKADER MAHAMMEDI, MD

SOMA SENGUPTA, MD, PHD, FRCP

The brain consists of four major lobes, known as the frontal, occipital, parietal, and temporal lobes. Each holds its very own distinct function and can be further categorized by which side of the brain it is located—right or left. Of the four, the temporal lobe is in closest proximity to the ears and contains the primary auditory cortex, which acts as the first stop for auditory information that is being processed by the brain.[1] In addition to hearing, the temporal lobe is responsible for visual processing, object recognition, and navigation abilities as it contains both the fusiform face area and para-hippocampal place area.[2,3] These areas are responsible for recognizing faces and encoding information obtained from the visible environment, forming spatial memory.[4,5] As such, the temporal lobe is extremely important in terms of visual processing.

Wernicke's area is also located in the temporal lobe. It is responsible for language development, including forming and comprehending verbal speech and language.[6] Specifically, the left temporal lobe is known for memory, speech, and behavior in comparison to the right temporal lobe. It is believed to play a role in behavior due to its ability to process emotion.[7] Most people are dominant in the left temporal lobe. Patients with damage to the nondominant right temporal lobe would begin to recognize side effects with learning; however, any trauma to the left temporal lobe could disrupt any of the essential operations discussed above.[8] Columbus's story is of a 55-year-old veteran who served during Operation Desert Storm. He developed significant spatial and speech challenges due to a glioblastoma discovered in his left temporal lobe. This is his story.

Columbus was known by his family, friends, and colleagues for his staunch dedication to military service and his meticulous work ethic. He was deployed to the Gulf War as a member of the Army National Guard, working to purify 100,000 gallons of water each day during Operation Desert Storm. His commitment to serving his country continued after his return. He joined an Air National Guard civil engineering squadron in Georgia that worked on humanitarian efforts like the redevelopment of a crumbling senior center in Armenia. However, it was during an extended assignment at the Pentagon in 2017 that Columbus first noticed something was wrong. After a long day, he began searching for his rental car in the parking lot. This simple task took him almost an hour. He finally called a coworker who informed him that the car was right in front of him. He jumped into the driver's seat only to find that he had no recollection of the hotel where he had been staying for nearly three weeks. Things only got worse when he got back from Washington D.C.; feelings of disorientation and an inability to recognize familiar places increased. He wondered why his memory and sense of navigation were declining. He decided to pay a visit to the doctor.

Columbus was slated to deploy in early 2018, but his military physician, assuming that his "brain fog" and correlating high blood sugar levels were due to diabetes mellitus, sidelined him in November of 2017. With a diabetes diagnosis and advice to cut carbohydrates in hand, Columbus kept working, but his struggles with short-term memory continued for months. By May of 2018, his symptoms had hit a critical level. Though he became adept at compensating for his increasing cognitive losses, his colleagues began to notice abnormalities in his written correspondence. He seemed to be having difficulty understanding language. Though this shift in communication may have been imperceptible to a stranger, it was obvious to his commander, who was accustomed to his meticulous approach to work.

Something was especially amiss on an ordinary May afternoon in 2018, prompting his commander to walk him straight to the doctor herself: a move that saved his life. On May 31, Columbus's physician received brain imaging that revealed the Grade IV glioblastoma multiforme (GBM) within Columbus's left temporal lobe and immediately arranged to have him travel two hours north to an Atlanta hospital via military escort. Of all the classifications of gliomas, World Health Organization (WHO) Grade IV is the most malignant, the most aggressive, and the most infiltrative; spreading the fastest into other areas of the brain, though it is very rare that the spread of this type of glioma extends outside of the brain. Additionally, as with Columbus, the GBM was classified as isocitrate dehydrogenase wildtype (IDH WT), which is far more aggressive that the alternative IDH-mutant. Columbus's case was so severe that Dr. Nelson Oyesiku, a neurosurgeon at Atlanta's Emory University Hospital, delayed his travel plans to perform a six-hour gross total resection surgery of the tumor within hours of Columbus's arrival at the hospital.

After the initial resection surgery, Columbus enrolled in a clinical trial at the Winship Cancer Institute at Emory in Atlanta with the help of Dr. Soma Sengupta. This trial tested the effects of the chemotherapeutic drug, belinostat, in combination with radiation and traditional chemotherapy. Belinostat is an intravenously (IV) administered histone deacetylase (HDAC) inhibitor and anti-cancer agent. It functions by blocking the HDAC enzymes, preventing histone proteins from playing their role in gene regulation, thus interfering with the genetic makeup of the cancer cells and ultimately leading to cell death. Upon the completion of his radiation therapy, he was given cycles of the alkylating agent Temodar, another antineoplastic chemotherapy treatment, along with the Optune® device, which he was prescribed to use for 18 hours each day. The Optune® device is both wearable and portable, consisting of transducer arrays that adhere to the skull and an electric field generator that Columbus carried in a backpack

throughout the day. The device resembles a thin white cap. The Optune®
device functions by delivering tumor treating fields (TTFs) via ceramic discs
within the transducer arrays which stick directly onto the scalp. These low
intensity, alternating electrical fields work not only to slow but oftentimes
to stop the growth and division of GBM cells by sending signals into the
brain to "confuse" the cancer. The Optune® device helps to increase the
lifespan of its users, like Columbus, for whom it was successful in attain-
ing such results. For many months, he was showing consistent compliance
with this treatment, ensuring that he used it exactly as recommended to
reap the greatest possible benefit from it.

Throughout the initial portion of the year immediately after the removal
of the GBM from his left temporal lobe, Columbus was asymptomatic and
independent in many of his regular day-to-day activities. This granted him
the freedom to pursue his lifelong aspiration of becoming an artist. He had
shied away from this dream when he was young, deciding instead to serve
his country by joining the Army National Guard, and later the Air National
Guard, where he served for a collective 30 years. He also continued his
work in the private sector as an architectural illustrator.

The cancer diagnosis only fueled his zest for life and creativity; his passion for art was revitalized. Inspired by Leonardo da Vinci, he had always
painted portraits and landscapes of notable places and people, such as
those he had encountered while serving in Operation Desert Storm. However, through his new lens on life, he began to construct large-scale mixed
media work, even incorporating recyclable parts of his Optune® device.

Unfortunately, an MRI scan in October of 2019 revealed worrisome
imaging of potential local progression of the tumor (Fig. 2.1–2.3). In
addition to this troubling discovery, abnormalities in Columbus's neurocognitive capacity, such as issues with his memory and word-finding capa-
bilities, were gradually becoming more pronounced. This word-finding
difficulty showcased itself through his inability to retrieve words for use
in regular speech, despite his retention of the ability to understand the
English language. To treat these new symptoms, Columbus was put on the
steroid dexamethasone.

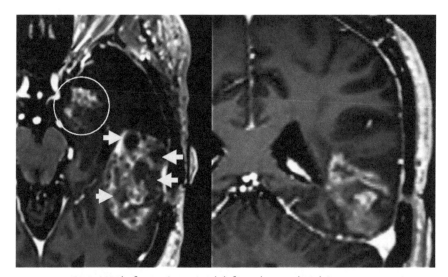

FIGURE 2.1   Brain MRI before surgery. Axial (left) and coronal (right) post-contrast images show a large mass that appears bright after being injected with IV contrast within the posterior and anterior aspect of the left temporal lobe (yellow arrows and circle), most consistent with high-grade glioma.

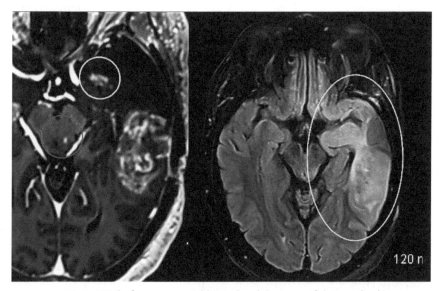

FIGURE 2.2   Brain MRI before surgery. Additional nodular areas of abnormal enhancement that appear bright after being injected with IV contrast are noted in the anterior temporal lobe (yellow circle) and the left aspect of the midbrain (red circle). There is surrounding signal alteration on the MRI sequence image most consistent with swelling (yellow oval).

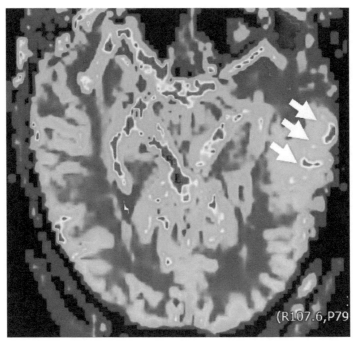

FIGURE 2.3   Brain MRI before surgery. Further exploration with advanced perfusion MRI demonstrates that this mass contains areas of moderately increased cerebral blood volume (CBV) (white arrow) suggestive of a tumor.

On February 25, 2020, Columbus underwent his second resection at the Dana Farber National Cancer Institute in Boston. Within two months of this procedure, the postoperative site had healed, and he began a combination of the Optune® device and Keytruda immunotherapy. The Keytruda treatment differed significantly in its mechanism from the traditional chemotherapy and radiation therapy that he had been prescribed prior. Keytruda works congruently with the immune system, specifically acting on the system's PD-1/PD-L1 inhibitory pathway to aid the body in fighting cancer. When functioning normally, the immune system uses T-cells, which act in detecting and removing abnormal cells from the body. Cancerous cells outwit this system by utilizing the PD-1/PD-L1 pathway, which allows them to hide from the T-cells and avoid being destroyed. Keytruda's mechanism is to block this PD-1/PD-L1 pathway, allowing the T-cells to once more regain the ability to do their job, ultimately terminating the cancer cells.

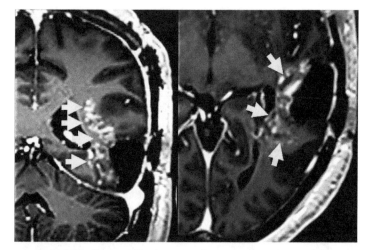

FIGURE 2.4   Brain MRI after surgery. Imaging shows post-treatment and post-operative changes from resection of the left temporal tumor. There are patchy and irregular areas of abnormal enhancement within the medial margin of the surgical cavity that appear bright after being injected with IV contrast (yellow arrows), uncertain for residual tumor versus post-treatment changes.

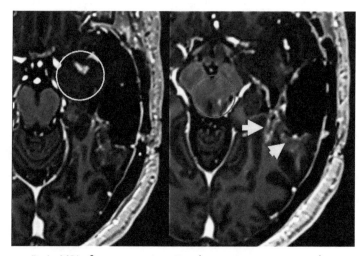

FIGURE 2.5   Brain MRI after surgery. Imaging shows post-treatment and post-operative changes from resection of the left temporal tumor. There is interval decreased abnormal patchy enhancement within the medial left temporal lobe (yellow circle) and stable tiny enhancing lesion within the left aspect of the midbrain (red circle), which are also uncertain for residual tumor versus post-treatment changes.

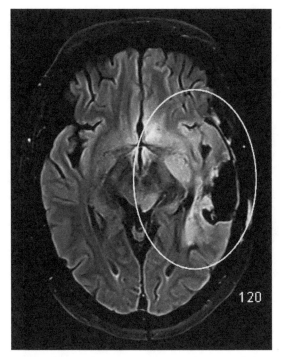

FIGURE 2.6   Brain MRI after surgery. There is surrounding signal alteration on the MRI sequence image similar to the MRI before the surgery, which is nonspecific but likely represents swelling (yellow oval).

Initially, after the treatment, there was no obvious progression in his symptoms, but by mid-May of that same year, there was a dramatic decline in his condition (Fig. 2.4–2.7). Several concerning transient symptoms appeared, including confusion, lethargy, and significant memory loss, which impacted his compliance with his treatments and caused him to sometimes forget his regimen.

Columbus's journey to recovery had been long, convoluted, and arduous, but he did not allow his challenges to break his stride. Following his initial resection surgery, he had to relearn simple tactile skills such as holding a pencil, writing, and drawing, and still, his optimistic demeanor persisted. Since the discovery of his GBM, after which he was told he had nine to 14 months to live, his family noticed very positive changes in his overall attitude toward life and a reinvigoration in his passion for art. As a

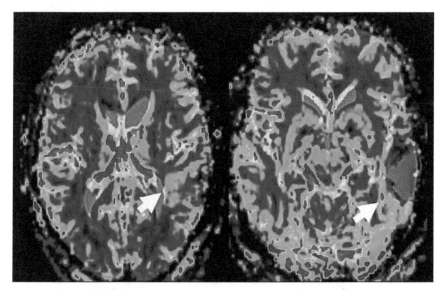

FIGURE 2.7 Brain MRI after surgery. Further exploration with advanced perfusion MRI shows a small focus of slightly increased cerebral blood volume (white arrow) which suggests that the majority of the abnormal enhancement is related to post-treatment changes with a small focus of residual tumor.

young man (Fig. 2.8), his laser focus on his career and service had drawn him away from prioritizing such self-expression. However, after his cancer diagnosis, his military friends and colleagues helped him build an art studio, where he was able to use his talent to create abstract art. He continued to paint, despite developing chronic visual abnormalities that inhibited his ability to drive.

Despite his constant battle with brain cancer, Columbus sustained his role as a dedicated father and devoted husband to his wife, Val, who was integral to his treatment and recovery journey. Columbus and Val, along with his physicians, decided to complement his use of Optune® and Keytruda with the chemotherapy drug Avastin in hopes to target the cancer cells more directly. Generically known as bevacizumab, Avastin functions in an anti-angiogenic manner, blocking the vascular endothelial growth factor protein (VEGF), preventing blood vessels from reaching and feeding the tumor. This ultimately results in starving the tumor and inhibiting its

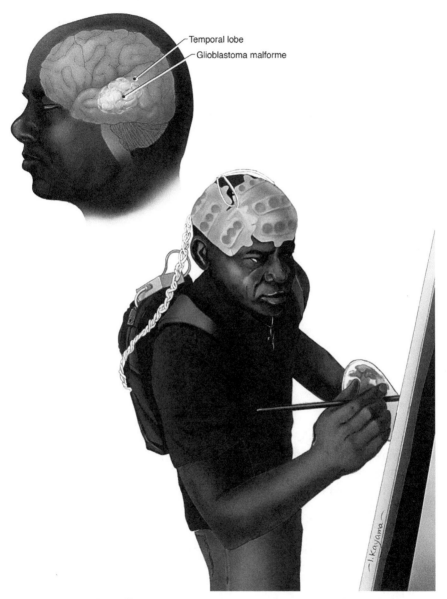

Temporal lobe
Glioblastoma malforme

FIGURE 2.8 (medical illustration) Columbus was diagnosed with a Glioblastoma multiforme (GBM) in the left temporal lobe of his brain. As part of his treatment, he wore an Optune device that delivers electric fields to the tumor site and interrupts cell division. Columbus had a passion for art and created many abstract pieces.

growth. Columbus continued with this combination for approximately six months. However, as 2020 came to a close, Columbus's GBM had a fibroblast growth factor receptor (FGFR) mutation. After discussing the strategy with Dr. Sengupta, Columbus's oncologist at Emory, Dr. Steven Szabo, decided to put him on Balversa. Columbus continued his treatments until March of 2021, when he passed away, still optimistic, kind, and grateful for the lessons of his journey until the very end. His legacy carries on through his wife, children, and scores of friends who dearly miss him. The Healing Arts Program at The Hudgens Center for Art and Learning in Duluth, Georgia, where Columbus had his first solo exhibition in 2019, will be named in his honor.

ENDNOTES

1. Dale Purves et al., *Neuroscience*, 2nd ed. (Sunderland, MA: Sinauer Associates, 2001), https://www.ncbi.nlm.nih.gov/books/NBK10900/.

2. Jeffery R. Binder et al., "Temporal Lobe Regions Essential for Reserved Picture Naming after Left Temporal Epilepsy Surgery," *Epilepsia* 61, no. 9 (September 2020): 1939–48. https://doi.org/10.1111/epi.16643.

3. Anand Patel, Grace Marie Nicole R. Biso, and James B. Fowler, "Neuroanatomy, Temporal Lobe," in *StatPearls* (Treasure Island, FL: StatPearls Publishing, 2021), http://www.ncbi.nlm.nih.gov/books/NBK519512/.

4. Jeffery R. Binder et al., "Temporal Lobe Regions Essential for Reserved Picture Naming after Left Temporal Epilepsy Surgery."

5. Anand Patel, Grace Marie Nicole R. Biso, and James B. Fowler, "Neuroanatomy, Temporal Lobe."

6. Jeffery R. Binder et al., "Temporal Lobe Regions Essential for Reserved Picture Naming after Left Temporal Epilepsy Surgery."

7. Ibid.

8. "Brain Map: Temporal Lobes," *Queensland Health*, Queensland Government, January 22, 2021. https://www.health.qld.gov.au/abios/asp/btemporal_lobes.

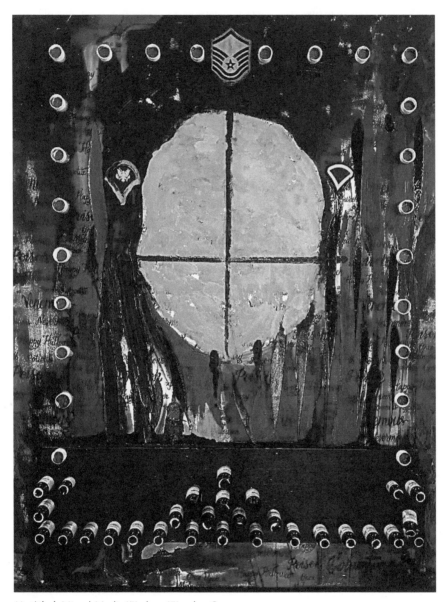

Untitled, Mixed Media Work on Wooden Canvas
(Acrylic, Broadcloth & Chemotherapy Vials)
by Columbus Cook
from the Collection of Columbus Cook Holdings

REFERENCES

Binder, Jeffrey R., Jia-Qing Tong, Sara B. Pillay, Lisa L. Conant, Colin J. Humphries, Manoj Raghavan, Wade M. Mueller, Robyn M. Busch, Linda Allen, William L. Gross, Christopher T. Anderson, Chad E. Carlson, Mark J. Lowe, John T. Langfitt, Madalina E. Tivarus, Daniel L. Drane, David W. Loring, Monica Jacobs, Victoria L. Morgan, Jane B. Allendorfer, Jerzy P. Szaflarski, Leonardo Bonilh, Susan Bookheimer, Thomas Grabowski, Jennifer Vannest, and Sara J. Swanson, fMRI in Anterior Temporal Epilepsy Surgery (FATES) study. "Temporal Lobe Regions Essential for Reserved Picture Naming after Left Temporal Epilepsy Surgery." *Epilepsia* 61, no. 9 (September 2020): 1939–48. https://doi.org/10.1111/epi.16643.

"Brain Map: Temporal Lobes." *Queensland Health*. Queensland Government, January 22, 2021. https://www.health.qld.gov.au/abios/asp/btemporal_lobes.

Patel, Anand, Grace Marie Nicole R. Biso, and James B. Fowler. "Neuroanatomy, Temporal Lobe." In *StatPearls*. Treasure Island, FL: StatPearls Publishing, 2021. http://www.ncbi.nlm.nih.gov/books/NBK519512/.

Purves, Dale, George J. Augustine, David Fitzpatrick, Lawrence C. Katz, Anthony-Samuel LaMantia, James O. McNamara, and S. Mark Williams. *Neuroscience*, 2nd ed. Sunderland, MA: Sinauer Associates, 2001. https://www.ncbi.nlm.nih.gov/books/NBK10900/.

CHAPTER 3

RIGHT TEMPORAL LOBE
The Woman Who Could Not Quench Her Thirst

ABIGAIL KOEHLER, BS

ROHAN RAO, BS

EASHIKA CHAKRABORTY

ABDELKADER MAHAMMEDI, MD

SOMA SENGUPTA, MD, PHD, FRCP

The cerebral cortex is divided into four major lobes based on their location within the brain. These divisions allow for neuroanatomists to subclassify groups of functionally related neurons, such as those of Broca's area and the primary motor cortex, based on their lobe location. In this case, the patient presented with a glioblastoma multiforme (GBM) in the right posterior temporal lobe. The gold standard treatment for a GBM is resection and chemoradiation, followed by the adjuvant chemotherapy drug temozolomide (TMZ).[1] GBMs can arise in multiple locations throughout the brain, but in this chapter, the temporal lobe was specifically affected.

The temporal lobe portion of the brain is located near the exterior structure of the ears and temple regions.[2] The outer surface of the temporal lobe is called the neocortex and contains the primary auditory cortex which is critical to the processing of sound.[3] Given the temporal lobe's close association with the other lobes, it also carries communication tracts to other parts of the brain. Thus, it is difficult to fully classify all the modalities with which the temporal lobe is involved. The inner surface, also known as the limbic cortex, includes the parahippocampal gyrus, hippocampus, and amygdala.[4] The hippocampus has been linked to memory formation and the amygdala is involved in emotional processing. Any damage impacting the hippocampus by the growing mass (mass effect) can lead to memory difficulties.[5] Insult to the amygdala will frequently lead to emotional and behavioral alterations. Auditory impairment can be a result of a lesion in the primary auditory cortex. Urinary incontinence is a common presenting symptom of brain tumors as it is usually the first symptom noticed by patients.[6] This is the story of Janet, who battled cancer for the second time in her life. Janet had many insights into working through cancer diagnoses; we will dive into her journey below.

Janet was 17 years old when she started college at Niagara University in New York to become a nurse. It was at this time when she received the terrifying diagnosis of stage IV ovarian cancer. A persistent fighter, Janet prepared herself for the long journey of battling cancer and overcoming it. At the time, Janet felt an overwhelming sense of inadequacy because her diagnosis was not something she could control herself; she could not stop it, she could not help it, and she could not make it better. She traveled to Memorial Sloan Kettering Cancer Center in New York once a month for chemotherapy treatment against her physician's opinion to get treatment once a week to maintain her academic status. Janet recalled her experience with treatment as awful. She was sick and in pain, all while juggling the hectic schedule of a nursing school student and young adult. She was ultimately rid of disease when she received a hysterectomy, including the removal of her cancerous ovaries. One can imagine the feeling of relief and liberation Janet felt when she no longer had to endure the pain and suffering associated with her cancer diagnosis.

One can also imagine why she would ask herself such a painstaking question, "Why me?", when she received a (GBM) diagnosis at the age of 66. Janet noted an intense thirst and painful, persistent urination in May of 2017. These symptoms prompted her to visit her primary care physician. Suspicious Janet might have of an overactive bladder or diabetes insipidus, which is characterized by chronic thirst and urination due to an imbalance of fluids within the body, her physician sent her in for imaging. On June 24th, 2017, however, her life would change forever. Janet's imaging showed a right posterior temporal brain lesion that indicated the existence of a GBM (Fig. 3.1). This location falls on the right side of the head, in the back portion of the brain, synonymous with the location behind the ear. She thought, "I had [cancer] once, I shouldn't have it again". She later underwent extensive

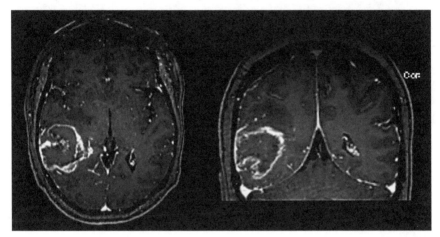

FIGURE 3.1   Brain MRI before surgery. Axial (left) and coronal (right) post-contrast images show a large mass centered in the right posterior temporal lobe with peripheral and irregular enhancement that appears bright after being injected with IV contrast, consistent with glioblastoma.

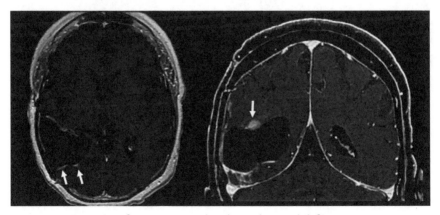

FIGURE 3.2   Brain MRI after surgery. Axial (right) and coronal (left) post-contrast images show postoperative changes from resection of the mass. Follow-up post-contrast images, obtained 29 months follow-up, demonstrate new nodular areas of abnormal enhancement that appear bright after being injected with IV contrast, along the superior and anterolateral margins of the resection cavity (white arrows), concerning for recurrent tumor.

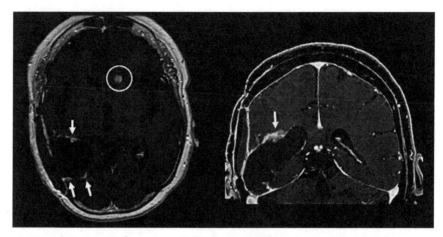

FIGURE 3.3   Brain MRI after surgery. Follow-up axial (left) and coronal (right) post-contrast images, obtained 34 months follow-up, show progressive increased size of nodular areas of abnormal enhancement that appear bright after being injected with IV contrast, along the superior and anterolateral margins of the resection cavity (white arrows), with a new abnormal ependymal enhancing nodule in the left frontal horn (white circle), concerning for recurrent tumor.

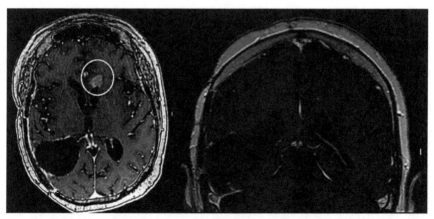

FIGURE 3.4   Brain MRI after surgery. Follow-up axial (left) and coronal (right) post-contrast images, obtained 39 months follow-up, show progressive increased size of an abnormal ependymal enhancing nodule in the left frontal horn (white circle) that appears bright after being injected with IV contrast, consistent with a recurrent tumor.

surgery to resect the tumor. The tumor was analyzed by pathologists at Emory, who shared it was O[6]-methylguanine-DNA methyltransferase (MGMT) methylated, epidermal growth factor receptor (EGFR) viii amplified, and isocitrate dehydrogenase 1 wild type (IDH-1 WT).

A month after her surgery, Janet began chemotherapy and radiation treatment. She began trialing different chemotherapy drugs recommended by her team of physicians to pinpoint which would be most effective for her tumor. She was unable to be treated with the standard-of-care drug, TMZ, due to a severe anaphylactic allergic reaction. Despite desensitization to try to ween her on TMZ use, she continued treatment with lomustine, a different chemotherapy drug. Janet was placed on multiple clinical trials starting with the Belinostat/MRSI (magnetic resonance spectroscopic imaging) study and later the 5-ALA (5-aminolevulinic acid) study. Early on in her treatment, Janet turned to tumor treating fields (TTFs), to see if that form of treatment could provide her the benefit of tumor reduction. TTFs are commonly used in the form of an Optune® device. An Optune® device is a physical, white-colored cap that patients can place over their shaved heads to reduce cancer cell growth through the electric fields that the device omits. In the fall of 2019, Janet moved her care from Emory University Hospital and Wake Forest Hospital to the University of Cincinnati Medical Center to follow her neuro-oncologist, Dr. Soma Sengupta, with whom she had formed a close relationship. Due to the progression of her disease Janet underwent a re-resection surgery in March of 2020 and was placed on the adjuvant letrozole drug study. She then started the chemotherapy drug bevacizumab and required stereotactic radiosurgery (SRS) for a new lesion (Fig. 3.2–3.4). She continued care through her doctors in Cincinnati in conjunction with the care she was receiving at Wake Forest Hospital. She felt prepared but nervous each time she underwent imaging because she knew if her tumor had grown, it would result in a change of course to her treatment.

Janet had a passion for music and played the guitar, ukulele, and harp (Fig. 3.5). Before the COVID-19 pandemic, Janet would play at music festivals, parks, or nearly anywhere she could get together with her former church worship leader. Music and religion supported her through many of her difficult times. She attributed nearly all her survivorship success to religion. Janet was also very passionate about jewelry making. Yet, Janet was completely frustrated with her physical abilities, which had been impacted by GBM. She noted weakness in her left side, mainly her shoulder, arm, and leg, which caused her to be unable to play music as she once did and be independently mobile. Janet struggled with balance and was unable to watch movies with complex plots due to her confusion and memory difficulty. She was also unable to control her bladder. Janet found herself unconvinced that doctors would ever be able to diagnose her incontinence because they were highly skilled and had not yet been able to do so.

As Janet continued her battle with GBM, she reflected on her relationships that supported her along her way. She often thanked her niece, who advocated for her brain tumor treatment and put her in contact with many extraordinary physicians who took tremendous care of her. She also recognized her loving husband of 48 years, as he was her primary caregiver, and drove her to Cincinnati, OH from their home in Zirconia, NC for treatment. Although she knew her family was scared to lose her, she appreciated their love and determination to help her get through her diagnosis. She also remembered her nurse navigator at Emory. She believed every cancer patient should have a nurse navigator to help direct patients through the difficulty of juggling an emotional diagnosis, different specialty doctor appointments, and treatment. Her advice to future brain tumor patients was: "Be straight up and honest with your doctors so they know what is happening."

Sadly, Janet passed away on May 23rd, 2021. She will be missed dearly by her loved ones. Janet was planning on writing two books about battling cancer: one from a patient perspective, and the other from a medical perspective by reflecting on her education and experience in the nursing field. She believed these would be helpful for future patients and those who interact with cancer patients.

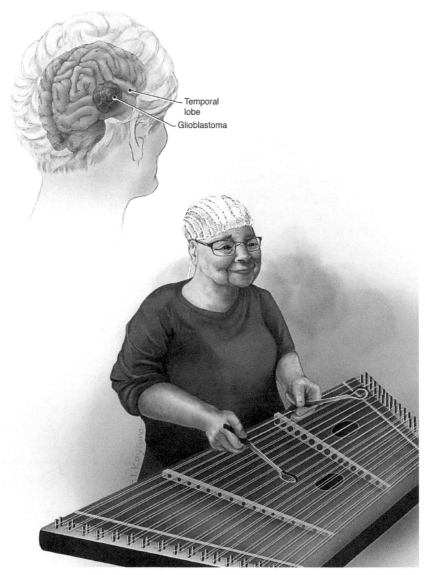

FIGURE 3.5   Janet was diagnosed with a glioblastoma multiforme (GBM) in her right temporal lobe. Janet enjoyed making music and playing different instruments. Here, Janet is playing the hammered dulcimer.

ENDNOTES

1. Roger Stupp et al., "Radiotherapy plus Concomitant and Adjuvant Temozolomide for Glioblastoma," *New England Journal of Medicine* 352, no. 10 (2005): 987–96. https://doi.org/10.1056/NEJMoa043330.
2. Anand Patel, Grace Marie Nicole R. Biso, and James B. Fowler, "Neuroanatomy, Temporal Lobe," in *StatPeals* (Treasure Island, FL: StatPearls Publishing, 2021), http://www.ncbi.nlm.nih.gov/books/NBK519512/.
3. J. A. Kiernan, "Anatomy of the Temporal Lobe," *Epilepsy Research and Treatment*, 2012 (March 29, 2012): 176157. https://doi.org/10.1155/2012/176157.
4. Michael J. Aminoff and Robert B. Daroff, *Encyclopedia of the Neurological Sciences, volume 1*, 2nd ed (London: Academic Press, 2014).
5. David E. Warren et al., "Medial Temporal Lobe Damage Impairs Representation of Simple Stimuli," *Frontiers in Human Neuroscience* 4 (May 18, 2010): 35, https://doi.org/10.3389/fnhum.2010.00035.
6. Leslie M. Okorji and Daniel T. Oberlin, "Lower Urinary Tract Symptoms Secondary to Mass Lesion of the Brain: A Case Report and Review of the Literature," *Urology Case Reports* 8 (June 4, 2016): 7–8, https://doi.org/10.1016/j.eucr.2016.05.005.

REFERENCES

Aminoff, Michael J. and Robert B. Daroff. *Encyclopedia of the Neurological Sciences, volume 1*, 2nd ed. London: Academic Press, 2014.

Kiernan, J. A. "Anatomy of the Temporal Lobe." *Epilepsy Research and Treatment*, 2012 (March 29, 2012): 176157. https://doi.org/10.1155/2012/176157.

Okorji, Leslie M. and Daniel T. Oberlin. "Lower Urinary Tract Symptoms Secondary to Mass Lesion of the Brain: A Case Report and Review of the Literature." *Urology Case Reports* 8 (June 4, 2016): 7–8. https://doi.org/10.1016/j.eucr.2016.05.005.

Patel, Anand, Grace Marie Nicole R. Biso, and James B. Fowler. "Neuroanatomy, Temporal Lobe." In *StatPearls*. Treasure Island, FL: StatPearls Publishing, 2021. http://www.ncbi.nlm.nih.gov/books/NBK519512/.

Stupp, Roger, Warren P. Mason, Martin J. van den Bent, Michael Weller, Barbara Fisher, Martin J.B. Taphoorn, Karl Belanger, Alba A. Brandes, Christine Marosi, Ulrich Bogdahn, Jürgen Curschmann, Robert C. Janzer, Samuel K. Ludwin, Thierry Gorlia, Anouk Allgeier, Denis Lacombe, J. Gregory Cairncross, Elizabeth Eisenhauer, and René O. Mirimanoff. "Radiotherapy plus Concomitant and Adjuvant Temozolomide for Glioblastoma." *New England Journal of Medicine* 352, no. 10 (2005): 987–96. https://doi.org/10.1056/NEJMoa043330.

Warren, David E., Melissa C. Duff, Daniel Tranel, Neal J. Cohen. "Medial Temporal Lobe Damage Impairs Representation of Simple Stimuli." *Frontiers in Human Neuroscience* 4 (May 18, 2010): 35. https://doi.org/10.3389/fnhum.2010.00035.

CHAPTER 4

FORAMEN MAGNUM AND HIGH CERVICAL CORD

The Woman with Rotating Paralysis

CHITRA KUMAR, BA

DANIEL MCGOUGH, MS

JONATHAN A. FORBES, MD

The lowest part of the brainstem is a structure called the medulla oblongata. At the transition between skull and cervical spine, also known as the craniocervical junction, the medulla oblongata transitions into the high cervical spinal cord. Both the medulla oblangata and cervical spinal cord are comprised of intricate sensory and motor highways responsible for transmission of information from the brain to the extremities. The "highways" in both regions are densely packed—as an example, the cervical spinal cord is roughly the same size as the human thumb. It is therefore no surprise that tumors compressing these structures can cause catastrophic neurologic dysfunction.

Neurofibromas are one such type of tumor that can result in compression of the high cervical spinal cord. The vast majority of neurofibromas, which arise from the sheath of peripheral nerves, are benign.[1] In many cases, neurofibromas are detected only after they have become large enough to compress neighboring neurologic structures.[2] Neurofibromas should be distinguished from schwannomas—a similar type of benign tumor that also arises from the peripheral nerve sheath.[3] The differentiation between neurofibroma and schwannoma is particularly important when surgical management is considered. Schwannomas tend to "displace" the parent nerve bundle and often can be easily dissected from associated nervous structures.

In contrast, neurofibromas often densely encase the associated peripheral nerve—placing this structure at increased risk when resection is chosen. As neurofibromas and schwannomas can have similar appearance on computerized tomography (CT) scans and magnetic resonance imaging (MRI), in many cases it can be difficult to differentiate between the two histopathologies prior to surgery.[4] It is important to remember that a small percentage of nerve sheath tumors can be malignant—this determination, which can only be made after microscopic evaluation of tumor tissue has been performed by the pathology team, can be critically important for delivering an accurate prognosis and selecting appropriate therapy.

As previoiusly discussed, neurofibromas and schwannomas arise from the sheath of *peripheral* nerves. However, when the site of origin is close to the *central* nervous system, it is possible for tumor growth to result in progressive compression of the spinal cord. As tumors initially compress the spinal cord, patients will often first note difficulty with balance secondary to early dysfunction of the posterior columns. As the degree of impingement progresses, it is common for patients to note some element of weakness, reflecting increasing dysfunction of the corticospinal tracts. Of critical importance, the corticospinal tracts consists of axons that carry information essential to movement from the cerebral cortex to the anterior horn of the spinal cord. After these impulses reach the anterior horn, peripheral nerves subsequently shuttle this information to the extremities.[5] Mild weakness secondary to early dysfunction of the corticospinal tracts can resolve completely following tumor resection. In patients with profound weakness prior to surgery, it is often not possible to restore complete function following tumor resection. When the tumor in question causes impingement of the high cervical spinal cord close to the region of foramen magnum, it is possible for patients to suffer a "rotating paralysis"—as experienced by our patient Isabella,* whose story we will discuss.

At 42 years of age, Isabella awoke one morning barely able to walk. This development was not surprising to her. Severe weakness predominantly

---

* a pseudonym

involving the left side of her body had been getting worse for half a decade. Initially, she had noticed mild problems with balance. Soon after, she began to have trouble picking things up with her left hand. Around this time, she immigrated with her 9-year-old daughter from her home country of Honduras to the United States. Following her arrival to the United States, Isabella began to notice that her left leg now appeared to be getting weaker. Weakness in her left arm had also clearly worsened—this extremity had become nearly useless for activities of daily living. As she tried to settle into her new job in the United States, Isabella found it challenging to manage her progressively worsening neurologic disability. She considered seeking medical advice, but as a Spanish-speaking immigrant with no health insurance and little in the way of a support system, she was hesitant to go to the hospital. The weakness on the left side of her body was getting worse. In addition, she had begun to note new weakness involving her right leg. Eventually, this weekness progressed to involve her right arm as well. When she awoke one morning barely able to get out of bed, Isabella knew there was no other choice but to seek medical care.

In the emergency department, MRI scans of Isabella's brain and cervical spine were obtained. MRI of the cervical spine revealed a large tumor near the craniocervical junction resulting in severe impingement of her spinal cord (Figure 4.1). The source of her progressive neurologic disability

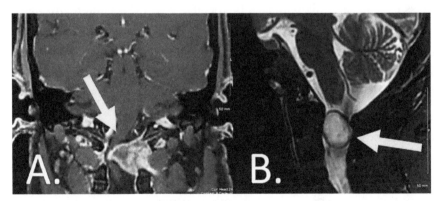

FIGURE 4.1   Coronal, T1-weighted, post-contrast (A) and sagittal, T2-weighted (B) imaging demonstrated a large extramedullary tumor (yellow arrows), resulting in severe impingement of the high cervical spinal cord.

had been identified. Based on its appearance on the MRI, the radiologist suspected the tumor was of peripheral nerve sheath origin

In the hospital, Isabella was introduced to Dr. Jonathan Forbes, a neurosurgeon specializing in tumors of the cranial base. During the first consultation, a muscle strength grading scale was used to evaluate the weakness in Isabella's extremities. This muscle strength grading scale ranges from zero to five, with a score of zero signifying a complete lack of muscle activation.[6] While some of her muscles scored a three or four, her entire left leg, from knee to foot, had no muscle activation and was scored 0/5. Her disability had progressed to the point where she dragged her left leg when attempting to walk. Her movements were ataxic, uncoordinated, and extremely labored. With the help of a translator, Dr. Forbes explained to Isabella that all her symptoms, from the weakness in her extremities to her difficulty balancing while walking, were a result of spinal cord compression caused by the growing tumor. He described the nature of the tumor and how, without intervention, it would likely progress with time to take away all remaining function in her arms and legs and possibly even her ability to breathe. The best course of action would be to surgically remove the tumor. After discussing the risks and benefits with her family and healthcare team, Isabella elected to proceed with the surgery.

The surgery was performed with Isabella in the prone position. Blood pressure was carefully managed by the anesthesia team and neuro monitoring was used to optimize safe perfusion of the impinged spinal cord during the tumor removal. Following exposure and boney removal, Dr. Forbes meticulously dissected the tumor free from the spinal cord under magnification and removed it without complication. A tissue sample was sent to pathology, confirming the tumor was a benign neurofibroma. Isabella did extremely well following the surgery. Shortly after the procedure, she began to notice the strength in her extremities was improving. At her one-year follow-up visit with Dr. Forbes, she had regained a great deal of strength and could even ambulate without using a cane. Repeat MR imaging did not show any evidence of residual or recurrent tumor tissue (Figure 4.2); other images showed that her spinal column remained perfectly

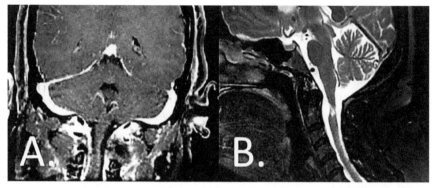

FIGURE 4.2 Coronal, T1-weighted, post-contrast (A) and sagittal, T2-weighted (B) imaging demonstrates no evidence of residual or recurrent tumor one year following resection. All mass effect has been relieved, and the spinal cord has re-expanded.

stable following tumor removal. At this visit, Isabella happily reported that she had recovered her ability to enjoy hikes and other outdoor activities with her young daughter for the first time in many years.

ENDNOTES

1. Lynn Messersmith and Kevin Krauland, "Neurofibroma," in StatPearls (Treasure Island, FL: StatPearls Publishing, 2021), http://www.ncbi.nlm.nih.gov/books/NBK539707/.

2. J.R. Leonard et al., "Cervical Cord Compression from Plexiform Neurofibromas in Neurofibromatosis 1," Journal of Neurology, Neurosurgery, and Psychiatry 78, no. 12 (December 2007): 1404–6. https://doi.org/10.1136/jnnp.2007.121509.

3. Miguel Esquivel-Miranda et al., "Anterior skull-base schwannoma," Neurocirugia (Asturias, Spain) 28, no. 6 (December 2017): 298–305. https://doi.org/10.1016/j.neucir.2017.04.002.

4. Rosalie Ferner et al., "Guidelines for the Diagnosis and Management of Individuals with Neurofibromatosis 1," Journal of Medical Genetics 44, no. 2 (February 2007): 81–88. https://doi.org/10.1136/jmg.2006.045906.

5. Adriana L. Natali, Vamsi Reddy, and Bruno Bordoni, "Neuroanatomy, Corticospinal Cord Tract," in StatPearls (Treasure Island, FL: StatPearls Publishing, 2021), http://www.ncbi.nlm.nih.gov/books/NBK535423/; Usker Naqvi and Andrew I. Sherman, "Muscle Strength Grading," in StatPearls (Treasure Island (FL): StatPearls Publishing, 2021), http://www.ncbi.nlm.nih.gov/books/NBK436008/.

6. Ibid.

REFERENCES

Esquivel-Miranda, Miguel, Elier De la O Ríos, Emmanuelle Vargas-Valenciano, and Eva Moreno-Medina. "[Anterior skull-base schwannoma]." *Neurocirugia (Asturias, Spain)* 28, no. 6 (December 2017): 298–305. https://doi.org/10.1016/j.neucir.2017.04.002.

Ferner, Rosalie E, Susan M Huson, Nick Thomas, Celia Moss, Harry Willshaw, D Gareth Evans, Meena Upadhyaya, et al. "Guidelines for the Diagnosis and Management of Individuals with Neurofibromatosis 1." *Journal of Medical Genetics* 44, no. 2 (February 2007): 81–88. https://doi.org/10.1136/jmg.2006.045906.

Leonard, J R, R E Ferner, N Thomas, and D H Gutmann. "Cervical Cord Compression from Plexiform Neurofibromas in Neurofibromatosis 1." *Journal of Neurology, Neurosurgery, and Psychiatry* 78, no. 12 (December 2007): 1404–6. https://doi.org/10.1136/jnnp.2007.121509.

Messersmith, Lynn, and Kevin Krauland. "Neurofibroma." In *StatPearls*. Treasure Island, FL: StatPearls Publishing, 2021. http://www.ncbi.nlm.nih.gov/books/NBK539707/.

Naqvi, Usker, and Andrew l Sherman. "Muscle Strength Grading." In *StatPearls*. Treasure Island, FL: StatPearls Publishing, 2021. http://www.ncbi.nlm.nih.gov/books/NBK436008/.

Natali, Adriana L., Vamsi Reddy, and Bruno Bordoni. "Neuroanatomy, Corticospinal Cord Tract." In *StatPearls*. Treasure Island, FL: StatPearls Publishing, 2021. http://www.ncbi.nlm.nih.gov/books/NBK535423/.

Waggoner, Darrel J., Jennifer Towbin, Gary Gottesman, and David H. Gutmann. "Clinic-Based Study of Plexiform Neurofibromas in Neurofibromatosis 1." *American Journal of Medical Genetics* 92, no. 2 (2000): 132–35. https://doi.org/10.1002/(SICI)1096-8628(20000515)92:2<132::AID-AJMG10>3.0.CO;2-6.

CHAPTER 5

BRAIN STEM

*The Nurse Who Started Having Double Vision
and Headaches*

ABIGAIL KOEHLER, BS

ROHAN RAO, BS

YANA TOMASSIAN

ABDELKADER MOHAMMEDI, MD

SOMA SENGUPTA, MD, PHD, FRCP

Regardless of location, many glioblastoma multiforme (GBM) patients experience painful side effects, such as headaches, due to increased pressure caused by the tumor mass.[1,2] Seizures are also common in GBM patients and are thought to be instigated by edema and neuroinflammation associated with expanding tumor.[3]

The left hemisphere of the brain contains many key areas associated with speech and motor movement. The major language centers within the left hemisphere include Broca's and Wernicke's areas. Broca's area is the premotor area for the coordination and production of speech, whereas Wernicke's area is connected with language comprehension. Aphasic symptoms, or the inability to create or understand speech, are typically caused by disruptions in the left hemisphere, as the major language processing centers are in this area. In addition to language and speech issues, motor issues can occur with insult to the motor cortex within the brain.

For most voluntary movement, the brain uses a two-neuron pathway that starts at the motor cortex and concludes at a target muscle to produce a given movement. The motor cortex in the left hemisphere is responsible for right-side movement, whereas the motor cortex in the right hemisphere is responsible for left-side movement. The brainstem also plays an important role in motor movement, as its primary role includes regulating balance and relaying motor movements to the rest of the body, among other things.[4]

This is the story of Beth, a young mother and pediatric oncology nurse who bravely battled a left cerebral GBM which ultimately metastasized to the brainstem.

Beth had a belated Christmas gathering with her beloved family over Martin Luther King, Jr. weekend in 2019. Beth was unusually quiet that weekend and had complained of severe headaches. Her primary care appointment was scheduled a few days later on January 23rd. At the appointment, her doctor scheduled her to see a neurologist the following week due to her excruciating headaches. As she drove home from the doctor, she had to stop the car multiple times to vomit. Upon hearing this, Beth's husband convinced her to let him take her to the emergency room (ER). In the emergency room, they did a computerized tomography (CT) scan and found a large tumor in the left hemisphere of her brain (Fig. 5.1). She was admitted to the hospital as the tumor would require surgery.

While Beth was admitted into the hospital, she had to wait until early the following week for surgery so that she could be medically stabilized. She had several visitors and spent time with her friends catching up and laughing together. One evening while she slept, she had her first seizure, which was notably long. Seizures were not a symptom Beth was anticipating, so it was incredibly scary for her and her family. After this seizure, she experienced aphasia, and she struggled to communicate with loved ones going forward.

Beth had a successful debulking surgery for her tumor. According to her surgeon, they were able to remove about 90% of the tumor, and it was sent for a biopsy to diagnose the type of cancer. The surgeon shared that it looked like a high-grade astrocytoma, but Beth's family stayed hopeful as Beth was young, active, and healthy. She was taken to the intensive care unit (ICU) while she recovered from surgery. The first day after surgery went well and she appeared to be making progress, but she fainted on the

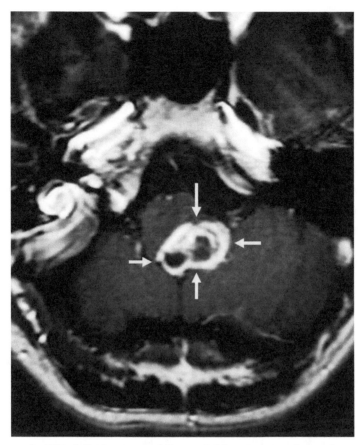

FIGURE 5.1   An MRI of glioblastoma multiforme. Axial post-contrast image demonstrates irregularly enhancing mass in the posterior aspect of the left pons extending to the fourth ventricle that appears bright after being injected with IV contrast (yellow arrows).

second day which extended her time in the ICU by few days. They hooked her up to the electroencephalogram (EEG) machine in the ICU to monitor after she fainted and seizures were detected. On day three, she was taken off the EEG when she had no signs of seizure activity. She was able to use her phone and read some messages, but the aphasia impacted her ability to write words and she was unable to respond. Beth felt frustrated because she was not able to speak or write what she wanted to communicate. Beth was discharged from the hospital on day four. At this point, only her speech was impacted by the tumor, so she was able to walk into her home and pick up her 13-month-old son, Sam. Both her son and her golden retriever, Spud, were extremely excited to have their mom home. She was doing well, both physically and emotionally, and was more worried about her parents and sisters than herself. This was typical of Beth, as she had been a bone marrow transplant nurse for children—she always put others before herself.

Beth started out-patient occupational therapy (OT) and speech therapy. Beth's aphasia continued to be a problem. Her initial speech therapy sessions were difficult as she became frustrated quickly when she could not come up with words. However, she continued to be positive and quickly learned ways to communicate when she could not come up with the words she wanted. Throughout Beth's journey, it was difficult for her husband to see people change how they communicated with her.

Following a confirmed diagnosis for GBM, Beth went on to see a neuro-oncologist, Dr. Soma Sengupta. Her diagnosis was very hard for Beth and her family to hear. However, Beth worked very hard to manage her aphasia, and she wrote the following message, "I'm thankful, but I'm worried too. I don't know what the future holds, but I know I love each of you." The plan was to start chemotherapy and radiation once the craniotomy scar had healed. However, Beth experienced a generalized tonic-clonic seizure and ended up back in the emergency room. While in the ER, she had another seizure on the way to get a CT scan, and she was admitted to the hospital. After she was held for observation for the day, they determined the seizures were caused by inflammation in her brain. Beth's steroid dosage and anti-seizure medication were increased, and she was released from the hospital later that day. However, after discharge, Beth had five focal or absence seizures. Her epileptologist increased the doses of her anti-seizure medication. This was a scary time for Beth, but she continued to be strong and enjoyed being with her family.

Beth had an appointment with her radiation oncology team later that week, but when she went home, her headaches worsened and her strong pain medication did not help, so she was taken to the ER again. She had a CT scan in the ER, and they found that her tumor had been bleeding which was causing pressure on her brain. While she was having the CT scan, Beth appeared to have a seizure and was not responsive. She was admitted into the ICU so that they could closely monitor her and do additional tests. Beth remained in the ICU and received the results of the magnetic resonance image (MRI) she had during the previous week. This showed that the tumor had almost fully grown back after her surgery, only 23 days before the imaging was taken. Beth was scheduled to start radiation and chemotherapy, but her care plan would have to be changed. The new plan was for Beth to have another surgery to debulk the tumor and "reset the clock".

Beth stayed in the ICU for observation ahead of the planned surgery. She had a few good days in the ICU, and she became more and more lucid as the week progressed. She was able to get out of bed a few times. Beth then had another successful surgery to debulk the tumor, just 31 days after her first surgery. They were able to remove a significant portion of the new growth, as well as a blood clot. Beth was moved back to the ICU after surgery to recover. She started to exhibit weakness on her right side after the second surgery and began working with the physical therapist to combat this. Her aphasia continued to worsen, and she continued to struggle to communicate. The plan was for her to be released to a rehabilitation hospital to begin radiation and chemotherapy. Unfortunately, she had a large, generalized tonic-clonic seizure that lasted over five minutes and was transferred back to the ICU. The large seizures seemed to knock out all her strength on her right side and she never regained much use or strength in her right arm and leg. During these challenging times, she continued to smile when she could and maintained a brave face for her parents, sisters, and friends.

Beth remained in the ICU and started chemoradiation as planned. Her friends, sisters, and co-workers decorated her radiation mask and painted it her favorite shade of blue, which made Beth smile when she saw it. Beth was also joyful when her son, Sam, was allowed to visit her in the ICU. He sat in the bed and just stared at her, smiling. She worked with physical and occupational therapy several times, but she was no longer strong enough on her right side to go to the rehabilitation hospital. She opted to have in-home rehabilitation.

The rest of the week and the following week went well with Beth continuing radiation and chemotherapy and enjoying being home. Spud, her dog, cuddled with her as often as possible, and Sam was thrilled to see his mom every day. Beth's mom moved in on the weekdays which allowed their family to get back into a routine. Beth's right-side weakness made it impossible for her to get around on her own and she was dependent on her husband to move her. The fatigue from radiation and getting in and out of the van each day were evident, but she remained positive.

Upon completing radiation, Beth rang the bell in her doctor's office, signifying she was done, with a huge smile on her face. Her radiation oncology team let her take home the mask that her friends decorated. Beth had her follow up with Dr. Sengupta to go over the chemotherapy plan, which included starting with Temodar five days on and then 23 days off. Beth and her husband asked about the fluid build-up they had noted, and she was instructed to discuss her concerns with her neurosurgeon. She received the results from her latest MRI which showed the tumor was consistent with the imaging after her latest surgery. She soon began chemotherapy. While at a follow-up with her neuro-oncologist, Beth had a focal seizure and went straight to the emergency room. The ER discovered that she had a urinary tract infection (UTI), and she was given antibiotics. The infection was also expected to be the cause of the seizures.

The swelling in her brain, also called hydrocephalus, continued to grow, and it became very painful for Beth. She underwent a third surgery to have a shunt placed to drain the hydrocephalus to her stomach.

Following her recovery from surgery, Beth had energy and was able to communicate better than she had been able to for a long time. She was happy and spent as much time as possible watching Sam play. She was even able to attend a church service, which she seemed to enjoy as she had not been able to get out of the house since she lost her strength on her right side. After continuous therapy, Beth was able to stand up for the first time since her second surgery. This made her friends and family extremely happy to see.

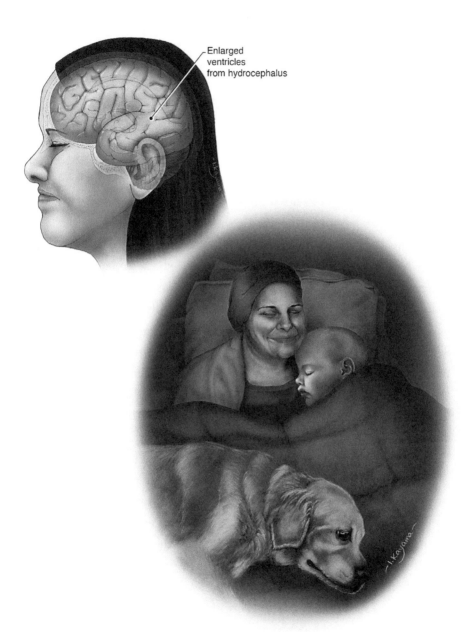

Enlarged
ventricles
from hydrocephalus

FIGURE 5.2 (medical illustration)   Beth had a glioblastoma multiforme (GBM) tumor in the left hemisphere of her brain that caused a buildup of fluid. Though she battled difficult side effects from her tumor, including pain from the swelling, she found comfort in spending time with her family, including her son, Sam, and her golden retriever, Spud.

Beth had an appointment with Optune® and started using their product. She also had a follow-up appointment with the radiation oncologist to go over the results of the MRI. The original tumor site was consistent, but there was a new spot in her brain stem that they were concerned with although they were not certain it was a new tumor. Her aphasia started becoming more of an issue and her strength was also starting to decrease noticeably. Beth's symptoms continued to worsen, and her appetite decreased as the week progressed. She started experiencing a lot of confusion as well. She ripped off the Optune® device multiple times throughout the week and did not seem to understand what it was. She was increasingly exhausted and slept more and more.

Beth became nauseous and was transported via ambulance to the emergency room. She had a very bad seizure that lasted around 10 minutes that night. She was not able to communicate verbally again after that and was mostly unresponsive. She had an MRI early the following morning which showed the spot on her brain stem was a tumor and had grown tremendously since the last MRI 15 days before. Based on the size, location, and aggressiveness of the new tumor, as well as Beth's deteriorating condition, her husband decided to discontinue treatment and start hospice care at home.

Beth was able to open her eyes to see her son and answer a follow-up phone call from her neuro-oncologist. She was able to communicate occasionally by squeezing with her left hand but was not able to open her eyes or speak again. It was the night of GBM Awareness Day, sponsored by the National Brain Tumor Society, in Washington, D.C. (July 20th) that Beth took her last breath. She was surrounded by her loved ones in her home. Beth was a truly incredible woman. She fought an unfair battle as hard as she could and did so with a smile on her face. Beth loved everyone she met and touched so many lives. Her husband later read in her blog from the time she spent in Uganda that she "had the honor curse of ushering several babies into heaven" during her time as a pediatric oncology nurse. Her husband believes that they were there waiting for her with open arms.

ENDNOTES

1. Dongyou Liu, *Tumors and Cancers: Central and Peripheral Nervous Systems* (Boca Raton, FL: CRC Press, 2018), https://doi.org/10.1201/9781315120522.

2. Robert Grant, "Overview: Brain Tumour Diagnosis and Management/Royal College of Physician Guidelines," *Journal of Neurology, Neurosurgery, and Psychiatry* 75, no. Suppl II (June 2004): 18–23. https://doi.org/10.1136/jnnp.2004.040360.

3. O. Prakash et al., "Gliomas and Seizures," *Medical Hypotheses* 79, no. 5 (November 2012): 622–26. https://doi.org/10.1016/j.mehy.2012.07.037.

4. Joel D. Swartz et al., "Balance and Equilibrium, II: The Retrovestibular Neural Pathway," *American Journal of Neuroradiology* 17, no. 6 (June 1996): 1187–90.

REFERENCES

Liu, Dongyou. *Tumors and Cancers: Central and Peripheral Nervous Systems*. Boca Raton, FL: CRC Press, 2018. https://doi.org/10.1201/9781315120522.

Grant, Robert. "Overview: Brain Tumour Diagnosis and Management/Royal College of Physician Guidelines." *Journal of Neurology, Neurosurgery, and Psychiatry* 75, no. Suppl 2 (June 2004): 18–23. https://doi.org/10.1136/jnnp.2004.040360.

Prakash, O., W.J. Lukiw, F. Peruzzi, K. Reiss, and A.E. Musto. "Gliomas and Seizures." *Medical Hypotheses* 79, no. 5 (November 2012): 622–26. https://doi.org/10.1016/j.mehy.2012.07.037.

Swartz, Joel D., David L. Daniels, H. Ric Harnsberger, John L. Ulmer, Steven Harvey, Katherine A. Shaffer, and Leighton Mark. "Balance and Equilibrium, II: The Retrovestibular Neural Pathway." *American Journal of Neuroradiology* 17, no. 6 (June 1996): 1187–90. http://www.ajnr.org/content/ajnr/17/6/1187.full.pdf.

CHAPTER 6

CEREBELLUM
The Woman with Pigmented Lesions and Worsening Balance

SHUSHMA GUDLA, BS
BRENDAN WILSON, PA-C
DANIEL MCGOUGH, MS
JONATHAN A. FORBES, MD

Neurofibromatosis type 1 (NF1) is the most common single gene disorder in humans, occurring in about 1 in 3,000 births worldwide. Patients who suffer from NF1 harbor a mutation in neurofibromin, a particularly large gene located on the long arm of chromosome 17. NF1 is one of the five main phakomatoses, which are rare genetic syndromes involving derivatives of the embryonic ectoderm—including the skin and nervous system. Common manifestations of NF1 include brownish spots in the iris known as Lisch nodules, rubbery masses in the skin and other regions of the body (which represent predominantly-benign nerve sheath tumors known as neurofibromas), freckling of the axillary or inguinal regions, and/or numerous flat, pigmented lesions of the skin called café au lait (meaning "coffee with milk") spots. Of particular importance, individuals affected with NF1 have much higher rates of cancer and cardiovascular disease than the general population, including a predisposition to develop glial tumors of the central nervous system (CNS). The cerebellum is one such structure in the CNS that can be affected.

The cerebellum serves to coordinate voluntary movements and bal-ance.[1] It receives signals that relay the position of the body and extremities in space and helps to integrate these signals with ongoing movement—facilitating smooth and controlled motor activity.[2] Generally speaking, the cerebellum can be divided into three functional regions. The central portion, or vermis, works with the flocculonodular lobe in coordination of vestibulo-ocular reflexes and regulation of muscles of the neck and trunk. Lesions involving either of these areas can result in uncoordinated movement of the head and trunk, problems with coordination of eye movements, and/or a type of gait instability known as truncal ataxia.[3] The region lateral to the vermis, also known as the intermediate zone of the cerebellar hemisphere, helps to regulate position sense and coordinate movements of the extremities. Lesions in this area can result in a phe-nomenon known as dysmetria, where individuals "undershoot" or "over-shoot" the intended position with the affected upper or lower extremity. Lesions of the intermediate zone of the cerebellum can also result in imbalance, often manifesting in affected individuals as falling towards the side of the lesion—as was the case with our patient Jane,* whose story we will discuss.[4] The most lateral portion of the cerebellum assists in the planning of sequential movements and conscious assessment of move-ment errors.[5] Unilateral lesions of the lateral cerebellum tend to be less symptomatic than lesions in the vermis or intermediate cerebellum.

Jane was 37 years old when she first noticed issues involving the left side of her body. In discussing this history months later, Jane was able to name the exact time and place she noted something was truly wrong. On a summer afternoon playing fetch with her dogs, Jane's left arm seemed to not want to work correctly. She tried not to think about the arm and hoped the symptoms would improve with time. Instead, in subsequent weeks, the sensation of clumsiness began also to involve her left leg and her balance. Soon after, she began to suffer from headaches that seemed to be worse in the early morning hours—prompting a visit with her

---

* a pseudonym

physician. In her doctor's office, Jane had difficulty touching her nose and then touching her physician's finger with her left hand—a sign of dysmetria of the left upper extremity. Abnormalities with balance were also noted when Jane was tested with tandem gait assessment. Aware of Jane's complex past medical history, her physician promptly ordered an MRI of the brain.

Jane had been diagnosed with NF1 at an early age after her pediatrician identified a number of skin findings, including café au lait spots. During these early visits, Jane's pediatrician had also noted she had trouble seeing out of her left eye. Imaging of the orbit and brain at this time demonstrated a tumor on Jane's optic nerve called an optic glioma, known to be found with increased frequency in patients with NF1. Jane recalls having eye surgery at a young age and wearing an eye patch for a few weeks. During high school, she was found to have scoliosis of the spine—also related to her history of NF1. She went on to graduate from college and found a job as an elementary school teacher. After marriage,

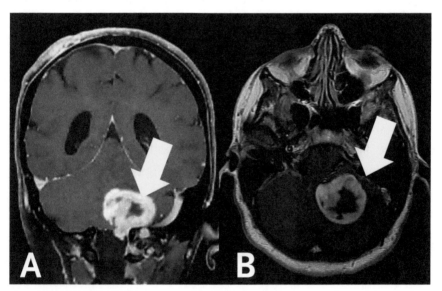

FIGURE 6.1   MRI of a Glioblastoma Multiforme. Pre-operative coronal (A) and sagittal (B) MRI demonstrates a mass with central cystic areas (yellow arrows) in the left cerebellar hemisphere.

Jane decided against having kids out of fear of passing on her genetic mutation. She had been well until that summer day playing fetch with her dogs.

The MRI ordered by Jane's physician demonstrated an enhancing lesion involving the intermediate zone of the left cerebellar hemisphere—suspicious for a type of malignant tumor of the brain known as a glioblastoma multiforme (GBM) (Figure 6.1).

Jane was referred to Dr. Jonathan Forbes, a neurosurgeon specializing in tumors of the brain and cranial base, for further evaluation. Dr. Forbes discussed the differential diagnosis. Radiographically, the tumor appeared to be most consistent with a type of cancer called glioblastoma (GBM), although GBMs were known to be uncommonly found in the cerebellum[6]. Specifically, the tumor was located in the inferior aspect of the left cerebellar hemisphere, with slight extension into the cerebello-medullary fissure. Jane's case was presented at brain tumor conference, where surgery was recommended. The risks, benefits, and expectations associated with the surgery were discussed in great detail. Jane agreed to proceed with surgery. In the surgery, Dr. Forbes removed a circle of bone overlying the cerebellum to gain access to the tumor (Figure 6.2). The boney removal was extended to the foramen magnum. Using neuro-monitoring and navigation, the tumor was meticulously dissected from the posterior inferior cerebellar artery and cranial nerves 9, 10, and 11 under high magnification. The tumor was removed without complication. Jane did well following the surgery and was discharged on post-operative day 3. Her immediate post-operative MRI demonstrated complete resection of the tumor without untoward finding. After the pathology returned consistent with GBM, Jane required treatment with radiation and multiple cycles of chemotherapy. A few weeks following surgery, all of her presenting symptoms were noted to have resolved.

The prognosis for GBM is generally poor—the median survival is roughly 12 months after diagnosis.[7] Incredibly, Jane has continued to defy all odds following the surgery. Her most recent MRI, now three and half

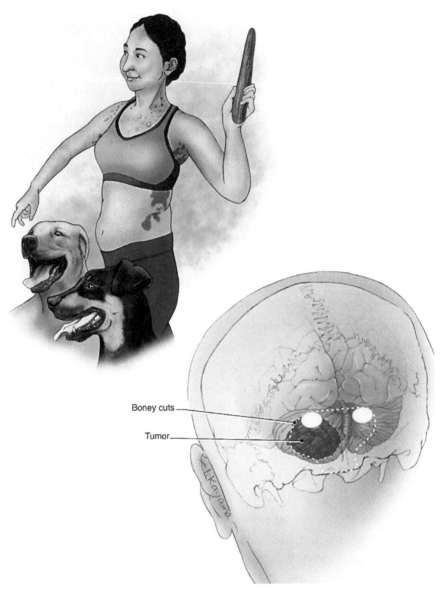

FIGURE 6.2 [Upper left] Jane first noticed clumsiness of her left arm on a summer afternoon while playing fetch with her dogs. [Bottom right] The boney cuts used to remove the tumor are outlined. The tumor was meticulously dissected from the posterior inferior cerebellar artery and CN 9-11 under high magnification and removed.

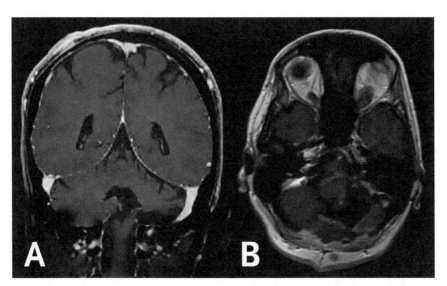

FIGURE 6.3 Two-year Follow-up MRI. Post-operative coronal (A) and sagittal (B) MRI continues to demonstrate no evidence of tumor recurrence following her original gross total resection.

years following the procedure, continues to demonstrate no evidence of any residual or recurrent tumor (Figure 6.3). As a cancer survivor, Jane continues in her courageous battle against NF1. Her determination in the face of adversity remains a source of inspiration for her friends, family members, and providers.

ENDNOTES

1. Ahmad Faleh Tamimi and Malik Juweid, "Epidemiology and Outcome of Glioblastoma," in *Glioblastoma*, ed. Steven De Vleeschouwer (Brisbane, Australia: Codon Publications, 2017), 143-153.
2. S. Jimsheleishvili and M. Dididze, "Neuroanatomy, Cerebellum," in *StatPearls* (Treasure Island, FL: StatPearls Publishing, 2021).
3. Ibid.
4. James A. Nelson and Erik Viirre, "The clinical differentiation of cerebellar infarction from common vertigo syndromes," *The Western Journal of Emergency Medicine* 10, 4 (2009): 273-7.
5. Ibid.
6. Ahmad Faleh Tamimi and Malik Juweid, "Epidemiology and Outcome of Glioblastoma," in *Glioblastoma*, ed. Steven De Vleeschouwer (Brisbane, Australia: Codon Publications, 2017), 143-153.
7. Monika E. Hegi et al., "MGMT Gene Silencing and Benefit from Temozolomide in Glioblastoma," *New England Journal of Medicine* 352, no. 10 (March 2005): 1000, https://doi.org/10.1056/nejmoa043331.

REFERENCES

Hegi, Monika E., Annie-Claire Diserens, Thierry Gorlia, Marie-France Hamou, Nicolas de Tribolet, Michael Weller, Johan M. Kros, Johannes A. Hainfellner, Warren Mason, Luigi Mariani, Jacoline E.C. Bromberg, Peter Hau, René O. Mirimanoff, J. Gregory Cairncross, Robert C. Janzer, and Roger Stupp. "MGMT Gene Silencing and Benefit from Temozolomide in Glioblastoma." *New England Journal of Medicine* 352, no. 10 (March 2005): 1000, https://doi.org/10.1056/nejmoa043331.

Jimsheleishvili, S. and M. Dididze, "Neuroanatomy, Cerebellum." In *StatPearls*. Treasure Island, FL: StatPearls Publishing, 2021.

Nelson, James A. and Erik Viirre, "The clinical differentiation of cerebellar infarction from common vertigo syndromes." *The Western Journal of Emergency Medicine* 10, 4 (2009): 273-7.

Tamimi, Ahmad Faleh and Malik Juweid. "Epidemiology and Outcome of Glioblastoma." In *Glioblastoma*, ed. Steven De Vleeschouwer. Brisbane, Australia: Codon Publications, 2017), 143-153.

CHAPTER 7

PITUITARY AND STALK

Visual Loss and Hormonal Alteration
in a Young Transgender Woman

A. SCOTT EMMERT, BS
BRENDAN WILSON, PA-C
AHMED HUSSEIN, MD
JONATHAN A. FORBES, MD

Note: In this chapter, the authors will refer to the patient by their preferred pronoun
and name throughout, even when discussing events that occurred pre-transition.

Craniopharyngiomas (CPA) are benign tumors that originate near the hypothalamic region, pituitary stalk, and pituitary gland.[1] As CPAs enlarge, mass effect from the tumor can cause several problems, including visual deterioration and hormonal imbalance. The most common form of visual deterioration in patients with CPA involves loss of vision in the outer halves of both eyes, referred to as bitemporal hemianopsia. CPAs that are symptomatic are often treated with surgical resection. Increasingly, neurosurgeons have come to favor use of a type of rod/lens camera known as an endoscope to improve visualization during surgical removal of CPAs through the endonasal corridor. While CPAs are benign tumors, they are notoriously prone to delayed recurrence after resection.

Doctors refer to the pituitary gland as the "master gland" because it controls so many functions in the body.[2] In particular, the pituitary gland helps regulate the body's metabolism, response to stress, musculoskeletal growth, sex drive and development, and fluid/electrolyte balance.[3] Deficiency in any one of the many pituitary hormones can have profound effects on a patient. This is especially true in pediatric patients, where the pituitary axes are especially integral to early development. The majority of CPAs are either found in children between the ages of five to 14 years old or in adults 50 to 74 years of age.[4] Because the population of transgender patients with CPA is relatively small, little is known about the effects of craniopharyngiomas on gender identity in transgender (trans) individuals, or those whose gender identity does not align with their assigned sex at birth. In this chapter, we describe the story of Arianna,* a 26-year-old transgender woman, who was found to have a CPA originating from her pituitary stalk and compressing her optic nerves, resulting in visual deterioration.

Arianna was assigned male at birth. She recalls a typical childhood growing up, where she played sports and liked to draw. In her teenage years, Arianna began to feel as if something about her was different. While her peers became interested in dating, Arianna notes that she never had much interest in sexual topics. Moreover, she remembers that when all the other boys her age began to grow facial and body hair, she had failed to develop many of these secondary sexual characteristics. As Arianna grew older, she began to feel her gender identity didn't align with her assigned gender. Ultimately, she decided to proceed with gender transition.

During Arianna's first visit with her family doctor to discuss her possible transition, the doctor sent off labs to evaluate levels of pituitary-related hormones in her bloodstream. At this time, it was discovered Arianna was producing abnormally low levels of testosterone. As a significant percentage of patients have naturally lower levels of testosterone, her physician did not feel the need to investigate this further. After a few weeks of counseling, Arianna began treatment with feminizing hormone replacement therapy as a part of her gender transition. This consisted of a daily oral regimen of estrogen (estradiol) and spironolactone, a testosterone blocker. Two months into hormone therapy, Arianna felt very happy with the changes that were occurring. Around this time, she found a steady job and met a man named

---

* a pseudonym

James, with whom she ultimately fell in. It was not until Arianna and James had moved in together that James began to notice that something was wrong with Arianna's vision. Specifically, Arianna always seemed to be running into walls, doorways, or other objects that should have appeared in her peripheral vision.

The tunnel vision progressed to blurriness that Arianna became more aware of. As James recalls, "Things got to the point where I would have to stand right in front of her just to get her to notice me." At a check-up with her optometrist, serious abnormalities in both visual fields and acuity were noted. Arianna was immediately referred to a neuro-ophthalmogist, where Humphrey visual fields confirmed progressive visual loss in the outer half of both eyes consistent with bitemporal hemianopsia (Figure 7.1).[5] An MRI scan of the brain was subsequently ordered. The MRI demonstrated an enhancing lesion involving the sellar and suprasellar regions with severe associated compression of the optic nerves and chiasm (Figure 7.2). The radiographic features of the tumor were most consistent with a craniopharyngioma.

Arianna was then referred to Dr. Jonathan Forbes, a neurosurgeon who specializes in tumors of the skull base. Dr. Forbes informed Arianna

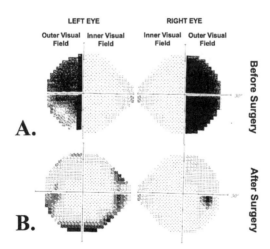

FIGURE 7.1   (A) Vision testing before surgery shows loss of vision (black shading) in the outer halves of both eyes. (B) Vision testing after surgery shows nearly complete restoration of vision (white areas) after full removal of the tumor. Black-shaded areas represent regions of vision loss, while white areas represent regions of normal vision.

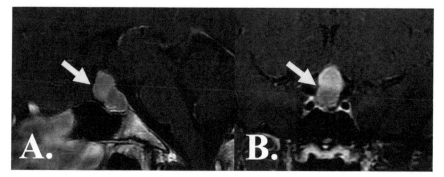

FIGURE 7.2   MRI of a Complex Craniopharyngioma of the Brain. Pre-operative MRI demonstrates a craniopharyngioma (yellow arrows) resulting in severe compression of important brain structures required for vision.

that her pituitary gland was not working correctly and she would need to be evaluated by an endocrinologist for supplementation of pituitary hormones. He also informed her that, following hormonal optimization, surgical removal of the tumor would be necessary to prevent additional visual deterioration. After the visit with Dr. Forbes, Arianna was seen by the endocrinology team, who acknowledged that the tumor may have been affecting the function of her pituitary gland for many years prior to her visual symptoms. Feeling better on medications prescribed by endocrinology, Arianna returned to Dr. Forbes' office to review the surgical plan in greater detail. During the surgery, a camera known as an endoscope would be passed into Arianna's nose to provide visualization (Figure 7.3). No external incisions would be used. Arianna was ready to proceed with the surgery.

On the day of the procedure, Dr. Forbes met Arianna and James in the pre-operative waiting area. In the operating room, the otolaryngology team performed the initial exposure and then turned over care to Dr. Forbes. After opening the leathery covering overlying the brain and optic nerves, Dr. Forbes identified the craniopharyngioma. He utilized high magnification with the endoscope to meticulously dissect the tumor from Arianna's optic nerves. The entire tumor could be removed. Arianna noticed an improvement in her vision almost immediately after awakening from anesthesia.

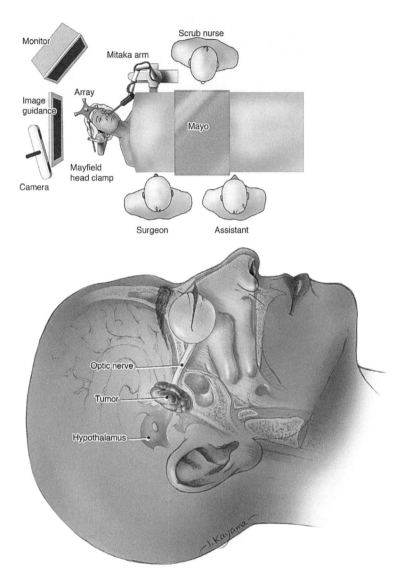

FIGURE 7.3 (medical illustration)   Artist's rendering of the surgical team and operating room during removal of a craniopharyngioma. Important components of the surgical set-up include equipment to position the patient (Mayfield head clamp), visualize the brain (camera, image guidance, monitor), and perform surgery (Mitaka arm, Mayo stand). The bottom image shows a magnified view of a craniopharyngioma (tumor) within the brain of a patient. Compression of important brain structures like the hypothalamus and optic nerve by the tumor causes changes in behavior, emotion, and vision that are characteristic of patients with craniopharyngioma.

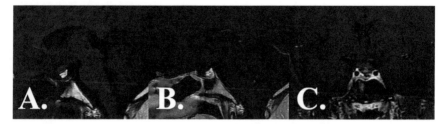

FIGURE 7.4   Post-operative MRI demonstrates complete removal of the tumor with no evidence of returning growth.

Arianna and her doctors have been very pleased with her recovery after the surgery. MRIs obtained at six months (Figure 7.4), and twelve months following the operation have shown no evidence of residual or recurrent tumor. Arianna's vision has been completely restored; all other symptoms have resolved under the care of the endocrinology team. She has been able to restart her hormone therapy regimen to reaffirm her identity as a transgender woman. After defeating struggles with identity, hormonal fluctuation, visual loss, and tumor removal, Arianna was ready to live life to its fullest.

ENDNOTES

1. Halil Tekiner, Niyazi Acer, and Fahrettin Kelestimur, "Sella Turcica: An Anatomical, Endocrinological, and Historical Perspective," *Pituitary* 18, no. 4 (2015): 575–78. https://doi.org/10.1007/s11102-014-0609-2.

2. Arun Paul Amar and Martin H. Weiss, "Pituitary Anatomy and Physiology," *Neurosurgery Clinics of North America* 14, no. 1 (January 2003): 11–23, v. https://doi.org/10.1016/s1042-3680(02)00017-7.

3. Ibid.

4. E.H. Nielsen et al., "Incidence of Craniopharyngioma in Denmark (n = 189) and Estimated World Incidence of Craniopharyngioma in Children and Adults," *Journal of Neuro-Oncology*, no. 104 (2011): 755–63. https://doi.org/10.1007/s11060-011-0540-6; Greta R. Bunin et al., "The Descriptive Epidemiology of Craniopharyngioma," *Journal of Neurosurgery*, no. 89 (1998): 547–51. https://doi.org/10.3171/jns.1998.89.4.0547.

5. D.M. Lefkowitz and R.M. Quencer, "Bitemporal Hemianopsia," *Journal of Clinical Neuro-Ophthalmology* 4, no. 3 (September 1984): 209–12.

REFERENCES

Amar, Arun Paul and Martin H. Weiss. "Pituitary Anatomy and Physiology." *Neurosurgery Clinics of North America* 14, no. 1 (January 2003): 11–23, v. https://doi.org /10.1016/s1042-3680(02)00017-7.

Baskin, David S., and Charles B. Wilson. "Surgical Management of Craniopharyngiomas: A Review." *Journal of Neurosurgery* 65 (1986): 22–27. https://doi.org/10.2176 /nmc.37.141.

Bunin, Greta R., Tanya S. Surawicz, Philip A. Witman, Susan Preston-Martin, Faith Davis, and Janet M. Bruner. "The Descriptive Epidemiology of Craniopharyngioma." *Journal of Neurosurgery*, no. 89 (1998): 547–51. https://doi.org/10.3171/jns .1998.89.4.0547.

Lefkowitz, D M, and R M Quencer. "Bitemporal Hemianopsia." *Journal of Clinical Neuro-Ophthalmology* 4, no. 3 (September 1984): 209–12.

Müller, Hermann L. "Childhood Craniopharyngioma-Current Concepts in Diagnosis, Therapy and Follow-Up." *Nature Reviews Endocrinology* 6, no. 11 (2010): 609–18. https://doi.org/10.1038/nrendo.2010.168.

Nielsen, E. H., U. Feldt-Rasmussen, L. Poulsgaard, L. Kristensen, J. Astrup, J. O. Jørgensen, P. Bjerre, et al. "Incidence of Craniopharyngioma in Denmark (n = 189) and Estimated World Incidence of Craniopharyngioma in Children and Adults." *Journal of Neuro-Oncology*, no. 104 (2011): 755–63. https://doi.org/10.1007/s11060-011-0540-6.

Reichlin, S. "Neuroendocrinology of the Pituitary Gland." *Toxicologic Pathology* 17, no. 2 (1989): 250–55. https://doi.org/10.1177/019262338901700203.

Tekiner, Halil, Niyazi Acer, and Fahrettin Kelestimur. "Sella Turcica: An Anatomical, Endocrinological, and Historical Perspective." *Pituitary* 18, no. 4 (2015): 575–78. https://doi.org/10.1007/s11102-014-0609-2.

FURTHER READING

Demorrow, Sharon. "Role of the Hypothalamic–Pituitary–Adrenal Axis in Health and Disease." *International Journal of Molecular Sciences* 19, no. 4 (2018). https://doi.org /10.3390/ijms19040986.

Emmert, A. Scott, Ahmed E. Hussein, Olesia Slobodian, Bryan Krueger, Ruchi Bhabhra, Matthew C. Hagen, Sarah Pickle, and Jonathan A. Forbes. "Case Report of Transgender Patient with Gonadotropic Dysfunction Secondary to Craniopharyngioma: Toward Improving Understanding of Biopsychosocial Dynamics of Gender Identity in Neurosurgical Care." *World Neurosurgery* 145 (2021): 448–53. https://doi.org /10.1016/j.wneu.2020.09.168.

Fisher, Alessandra D., Jiska Ristori, Girolamo Morelli, and Mario Maggi. "The Molecular Mechanisms of Sexual Orientation and Gender Identity." *Molecular and Cellular Endocrinology* 467 (2018): 3–13. https://doi.org/10.1016/j.mce.2017.08.008.

Forbes, Jonathan A., Edgar G. Ordóñez-rubiano, Hilarie C. Tomasiewicz, Matei A. Banu, Iyan Younus, Georgiana A. Dobri, C. Douglas Phillips, Ashutosh Kacker, Babacar Cisse, and Vijay K. Anand. "Endonasal Endoscopic Transsphenoidal Resection of Intrinsic Third Ventricular Craniopharyngioma: Surgical Results." *Journal of Neurosurgery* 131 (2019): 1152–62. https://doi.org/10.3171/2018.5.JNS18198.1152.

Irving, Amanda, and William B. Lehault. "Clinical Pearls of Gender-Affirming Hormone Therapy in Transgender Patients." *Mental Health Clinician* 7, no. 4 (2017): 164–67. https://doi.org/10.9740/mhc.2017.07.164.

Joukal, Marek. "Anatomy of the Human Visual Pathway." In *Homonymous Visual Field Defects*, edited by Karolína Skorkovská. Cham: Springer International Publishing, 2017, 1-16. https://doi.org/10.1007/978-3-319-52284-5_1.

Safer, Joshua D., and Vin Tangpricha. "Care of Transgender Persons." *New England Journal of Medicine* 381, no. 25 (2019): 2451–60. https://doi.org/10.1056/NEJMcp1903650.

CHAPTER 8

TUMOR AFFECTING HEARING
Trials and Tribulations

ABIGAIL KOEHLER, BS
ROHAN RAO, BS
EASHIKA CHAKRABORTY
ABDELKADER MAHAMMEDI, MD
RAVI N. SAMY, MD, FACS
SOMA SENGUPTA, MD, PHD, FRCP

Within the brain, there exist a collection of nerves that function to control the sensation and motor functions of the head. One of these is called the vestibulocochlear nerve or cranial nerve VIII (CN VIII), which receives balance and hearing information from the structures of the inner ear.[1] As with most nerves throughout the body, CN VIII is surrounded by a coating of fat, termed myelin, speeding its conduction of electrical signals. The myelin sheath has a role similar to the insulation surrounding typical copper wiring. Both myelin and this insulation serve to speed up the electrical conduction along the length of the neuron and copper wire, respectively. Within the nervous system, two cell types, oligodendrocytes and Schwann cells, function to produce this myelin and properly envelope the axons. Oligodendrocytes are primarily found within the head and spinal cord whereas Schwann cells are found in peripheral nerves which connect the head to the rest of the body.[2] As can be insinuated from the name of the disease, a vestibular schwannoma involves a growth of the Schwann cells involved in creating the myelin around CN VIII.

Vestibular schwannomas (VS), also known by the term acoustic neuroma, have an incidence of approximately 3 cases per 100,000 patients/year.[3,4] The characteristic symptoms of VS include loss of hearing, imbalance, and ringing in the affected ear.[5] These symptoms are caused by a compression of CN VIII due to the expanding VS. As the tumor progresses, it may impinge on surrounding neuroanatomical structures next to CN VIII. One such structure is the cerebellum which is next to CN VIII's connection in the brainstem. Consequently, late-stage VS can manifest with limb dyscoordination, termed ataxia, and a diminishment of hand-eye coordination, termed dysmetria. Like many other disease processes, VS can be caused by genetic disorders, specifically the neurofibromatosis type 2 (NF2) gene. NF2 is relatively rare and constitutes only 5% of all VS.[6] Bilateral VS is the defining characteristic of NF2.[7] Below is the story of Jess, a small-town sock-lover who had to travel across the United States to receive care for her aggressive, fast-growing vestibular schwannoma.

At the young age of 26, Jess learned what it was really like to be an advocate. Beginning as early as 2009, Jess noticed she began having headaches that felt like Charley horses in her head. Her hearing also seemed to become impaired, and everything sounded as if she were underwater. She scheduled an appointment to see her primary care physician, who suggested she had a sinus infection with fluid in her ears. She was prescribed a common antibiotic and sent home to rest and recover. The only issue was, after completing her antibiotic regimen, Jess still had symptoms. After visiting with her doctor again, she was referred to a dentist with the potential diagnosis of grinding her teeth in her sleep. However, her dentist did not see evidence of this. After weeks of pain and no answer, Jess suggested to her doctor that she believed she should get a magnetic resonance image (MRI). Jess underwent imaging with a sneaking suspicion that something was wrong. Her fears were confirmed when her doctor called her on the phone and asked her and her husband to stop by the office. Her doctor was in more shock than Jess as she broke the news that Jess had a brain tumor. (Fig. 8.1). Jess's gut instinct was correct; there was something else going on in her brain.

Her tumor was a result of a genetic disorder Jess never knew she had called neurofibromatosis type 2 (NF2). She was diagnosed with a vestibular schwannoma tumor on the left side of her brain, which was pushing on her brainstem and wound around bundles of nerves. Later on, her mom found out that Jess's biological father was diagnosed with NF2 with similar symptoms to Jess and later passed away from his condition. Jess's siblings were tested but none have the condition.

Jess's physician referred her to many different Kentucky doctors who would fall short of being her advocate, "I'm sorry Jess, but this tumor is too complex, too big." Jess found herself terrified for her future as five different doctors could not seem to help her. To her, it seemed as though it were time to go home and die. She thought about how complicated her situation must be if so many people who train for this kind of work were not able to help.

One major advocate in her corner pulled through for her. Jess's mom was unaccepting of the fact that no one would help her daughter. She contacted the House Ear Institute in Los Angeles, CA to recruit Dr. Derald Brackmann to perform her difficult surgery. He planned to additionally

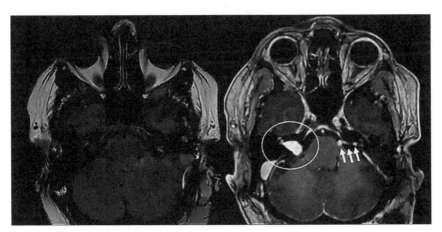

FIGURE 8.1   Axial images before (left) and after (right) injection of IV contrast demonstrate enhancing mass in the right internal auditory canal that appears bright after being injected with IV contrast (white circle), consistent with schwannoma. Post-surgical changes from schwannoma resection with persistent enhancement within the left cerebellar pontine angle cistern that appears bright after being injected with IV contrast (white arrows), consistent with residual tumor.

place an auditory brainstem implant (ABI). ABIs are surgically placed at the brainstem of a deaf patient and use an electrode to bypass damaged areas of the brain and create signals for the auditory nerve directly. Jess continued to work her job at a local bank up until the day she flew out to California. She felt very nervous but knew Dr. Brackmann was her only hope at combating her new diagnosis. Jess recalls the most difficult arrangement of her trip was figuring out who could take care of her dog! She expected to stay in California for 2-3 months, with 3-4 of the weeks in intensive care. Her entire surgery lasted 16-18 hours, but she was shocked when she woke and realized she only needed to spend about five hours in the intensive care unit (ICU). Unfortunately, she was unable to get the ABI due to her insurance denying her claim at the last minute. She stayed in LA for two weeks, staying in the hospital for only three days. She she did not need rehab or any other post-operative care. Jess remembers recognizing she was deaf in her left ear, but decided it was okay because she was alive.

Since there were not any physicians in Kentucky who could offer her treatment, Jess applied to the National Institute of Health (NIH) for a study. Jess thinks it is the craziest thing she has ever done in her life. She would hop on a plane to Washington, D.C. to receive chemotherapy, and fly back home. It was around this time that the tumor on her right side began to grow, and her hearing declined. She sought out Dr. Trent Hummel at Cincinnati Children's Hospital Medical Center, an expert in the field of central nervous system (CNS) tumors.

One day, however, Jess woke up completely deaf. Her hearing loss was later confirmed through the hearing tests she received regularly for following an Avastin chemotherapy protocol. Upon losing her hearing, she also lost her job. She was in touch with Dr. Ravi Samy, a neurotologist/skull base surgeon, at the University of Cincinnati Medical Center, for possible surgical treatment of her NF2. They discussed surgical removal of her tumors, radiation therapy, cochlear implantation, and placement of an ABI (Fig.8.1). Since Jess and her husband were unable to have biological children, they chose to adopt. She and her husband adopted two children who would play a significant role in Jess' treatment decisions. Although it was an uncertain time for her, she relied on her faith and family and ultimately decided that, despite the risks, "This may be a great opportunity to hear my kids for the first time." Subsequently, she underwent right-sided radio-surgery, a focused beam of radiation therapy, with her radiation oncologist, Dr. Luke Pater. Six weeks later, following the completion of her radiation therapy, she underwent cochlear implantation.

Before her implant, Jess read lips and communicated in sign language but found many barriers with this. When her cochlear implant was finally turned on, she heard her kids for the very first time. Later on, Dr. Samy informed Jess that she was still a candidate for the ABI during a follow-up appointment. He and Dr. Mario Zuccarello performed her ABI surgery at the University of Cincinnati and within six months she went from deafness to surround sound! Jess exceeded expectations with a 93% response to the ABI and, again, recovered quickly with no complications.

Throughout her journey, Jess has focused her attitude around two things: faith and crazy socks. Jess believes her faith carried her through her difficult journey and gave her a positive outlook on life. As for her love for crazy socks, Jess feels you cannot have a bad day if your feet are having a party! She claims she does not own any plain socks and her care team wears them during her treatment visits, follow-up appointments, and even her surgeries.

Jess's family is very supportive of her. Her husband was initially very worried about her condition and struggled not having answers or the ability to fix it. Her children grew up knowing about their mom's condition and understanding she was unable to hear them. Jess says that from the beginning she and her husband were very open with them about her condition. She brought them to doctor appointments, and they would sit with her while she received chemotherapy or watch through the window as she underwent radiation therapy. Jess loves to read and spend time with her kids as a stay-at-home mom. She volunteers at her children's school letting kids read to her. She also participates in Disability Day at their school by creating a mini station on the topic of deafness to educate children. She spends so much of her time advocating and educating that her young niece

FIGURE 8.2 (medical illustration)   Jess discovered she had Neurofibromatosis type 2 (NF2) after she was diagnosed with a vestibular schwannoma. The non-cancerous tumor was located near her auditory nerve and brainstem. Jess experienced hearing loss due to her tumor and eventually regained hearing with an auditory brainstem implant (ABI) and hearing aids. After all that she has experienced, Jess spends a lot of time educating young minds about the condition of deafness.

views her as a role model and sometimes wears a Cheeto behind her ear because it looks like Jess's hearing aid (Fig. 8.2).

Even through the most difficult times in her life, Jess has remained optimistic and thankful. Her advice to others who may be experiencing something like her situation would be to not stop just because someone else says you cannot do it. She reflects on her own self-advocacy, because if she had not asked for the initial MRI, her outcome may have been different. She also recommends keeping a positive attitude, saying "Life is so much better if you start looking for the good things instead of what could go wrong; think about what could go right. It's not 'I have to have,' it's 'I get to have.'" Jess personally only allows herself one day to cry and be upset, and then she reframes her attitude to match the motto she created for herself. Recently, Jess has scored a 98% on her follow-up hearing test, which is better than most people score. For Jess, life sounds good!

ENDNOTES

1. F.J. Laine and W.R. Smoker, "Anatomy of the Cranial Nerves," *Neuroimaging Clinics of North America Journal* 8, no. 1 (February 1998): 69–100.

2. J.L. Salzer and B. Zalc, "Myelination," *Current Biology* 26, no. 20 (October 2016): R971-R975. https://doi.org/10.1016/j.cub.2016.07.074.

3. Suvi Larjavaara et al., "Incidence of Gliomas by Anatomic Location," *Neuro-oncology* 9, no. 3 (2007): 319–25. https://doi.org/10.1215/15228517-2007-016.

4. Gino Cioffi et al., "Epidemiology of Vestibular Schwannoma in the United States, 2004-2016," *Neuro-Oncology Advances* 2, no. 1 (December 2020): vdaa135. https://doi.org/10.1093/noajnl/vdaa135.

5. Matthew L. Carlson and Michael J. Link, "Vestibular Schwannomas," *The New England Journal of Medicine* 384, no. 14 (April 8, 2021): 1335–48. https://doi.org/10.1056/NEJMra2020394.

6. Joshua Greene and Mohammed A. Al-Dhahir. "Acoustic Neuroma," in *StatPearls* (Treasure Island, FL: StatPearls Publishing, 2021), http://www.ncbi.nlm.nih.gov/books/NBK470177/.

7. Ashok R Asthagiri et al., "Neurofibromatosis Type 2," *Lancet* 373, no. 9679 (June 2009): 1974–86. https://doi.org/10.1016/s0140-6736(09)60259-2.

REFERENCES

Asthagiri, Ashok R., Dilys M. Parry, John A. Butman, H. Jeffrey Kim, Ekaterini T. Tsilou, Zhengping Zhuang, and Russell R. Lonser. "Neurofibromatosis Type 2." *Lancet* 373, no. 9679 (June 6, 2009): 1974–86. https://doi.org/10.1016/S0140-6736(09)60259-2.

Carlson, Matthew L. and Michael J Link. "Vestibular Schwannomas." *New England Journal of Medicine* 384, no. 14 (April 8, 2021): 1335–48. https://doi.org/10.1056/NEJMra2020394.

Cioffi, Gino, Debra N. Yeboa, Michael Kelly, Nirav Patil, Nauman Manzoor, Katie Greppin, Kailey Takaoka, Kristin Waite, Carol Kruchko, and Jill S. Barnholtz-Sloan. "Epidemiology of Vestibular Schwannoma in the United States, 2004-2016." *Neuro-oncology Advances* 2, no. 1 (December 2020). https://doi.org/10.1093/noajnl/vdaa135.

Greene, Joshua and Mohammed A. Al-Dhahir. "Acoustic Neuroma." In *StatPearls*. Treasure Island, FL: StatPearls Publishing, 2021. http://www.ncbi.nlm.nih.gov/books/NBK470177/.

Laine, F. J. and W. R. Smoker. "Anatomy of the Cranial Nerves." *Neuroimaging Clinics of North America* 8, no. 1 (February 1998): 69–100.

Larjavaara, Suvi, Riitta Mantyla, Tiina Salminen, Hannu Haapasalo, Jani Raitanen, Juha Jaaskelainen, and Anssi Auvinen. "Incidence of Gliomas by Anatomic Location." *Neuro-oncology* 9, no. 3 (2007): 319–25. https://doi.org/10.1215/15228517-2007-016.

Salzer, J.L. and B. Zalc. "Myelination." *Current Biology* 26, no. 20 (2016): PR971-R975. https://doi.org/10.1016/j.cub.2016.07.074.

CHAPTER 9

HYPOTHALAMUS AND THIRD VENTRICLE

The Woman Who Lost the Ability to Play Sudoku

DANIEL MCGOUGH, MS

CHITRA KUMAR, BA

JONATHAN A. FORBES, MD

The hypothalamus is one of the most fascinating regions of the human body. While it is one of the oldest and smallest regions of the brain (to be exact, the hypothalamus accounts for <1% of the overall mass of the brain), it is responsible for a number of diverse and critical actions. Important functions of the hypothalamus include regulation of energy metabolism and expenditure, fluid and electrolyte balance, sleep-wake cycles, pituitary function, breast feeding, body temperature, and arousal/wakefulness. Anatomically speaking, the hypothalamus is located below the thalamus and is bounded anteriorly by the optic chiasm. It is bordered laterally by the optic tracts and posteriorly by the mammillary bodies. In the coronal plane, the hypothalamus forms the walls of the third ventricle. With this latter relationship in mind, it is possible to understand why tumors occupying the confines of the third ventricle often manifest in hypothalamic dysfunction. Owing to its deep location and the functional eloquence of surrounding neurologic structures, a number of surgical approaches are often considered for removal of tumors involving third ventricle. These include, but are not limited to, the interhemispheric transcallosal, transcortical trans-choroidal fissure, subfrontal trans-lamina terminalis, and expanded endonasal approaches. Given the considerable risks associated with resection of tumors involving the third ventricle, the surgical approach must be meticulously tailored to the pathology at hand.

Tumors of the third ventricle are rare, accounting for between 0.6% and 0.9% of all intracranial tumors.[1] In general, tumors in this location can be classified as *primary* tumors, which arise from the immediate substance of the third ventricle (e.g. choroid plexus papillomas, ependymomas), or *secondary* tumors (e.g., craniopharyngiomas, optic nerve gliomas, hypothalamic glioma), that secondarily prolapse into the ventricle.[2] Chordoid gliomas are a very rare form of intraventricular tumor that sometimes arise in the third ventricle. Most of the known cases of chordoid glioma have occured in patients between 25 and 75 years old.[3] Of interest, there has been an observed 2:1 female to male ration in this cohort of patients. Individuals with chordoid gliomas can experience headaches, nausea, vomiting, endocrine disturbances, psychotic disorders, and/or visual deterioration.[4] In subsequent paragraphs, we discuss the story of Anne,* a 61-year-old woman who noted progressive worsening of vision, memory, and cognitive function. MRI imaging demonstrated a mass that would later be identified as a chordoid glioma in her third ventricle with severe associated inflammation of her hypothalamus and optic tract.

Anne was no stranger to health problems. Years earlier, she had been diagnosed with melanoma, the most serious form of skin cancer, in addition to several basal cell carcinomas. Although the melanoma was treated successfully with surgery, frequent reassessments with her physician team were required to ensure the cancer did not return. Both Anne's father and brother had been previously diagnosed with lung cancer. As a precautionary measure, Anne (herself a former smoker) had enrolled in a lung cancer screening program that annually assessed her risk with surveillance imaging. Anne suffered from a long history of cancer-related anxiety that had adversely affected her quality of life. This anxiety worsened when Anne began to develop new and troubling symptoms.

---

* a pseudonym

A lifelong fan of Sudoku, one day Anne noted that she was no longer able to solve puzzles that she would have easily breezed through in the past. In addition to these new issues with cognitive function, her vision and memory seemed also to be getting worse. Soon, other hobbies outside of Sudoku were affected. In seeking to reconcile these new and troubling symptoms, Anne initially tried to blame poor sleep or the normal aging process. Her husband ultimately helped her gather the strength to be evaluated by a doctor.

At the ophthalmologist's office, Anne described the feeling that objects were "jumping in and out" of her vision. Often, she felt as if she were "looking at the world through pinholes in a piece of cardboard." Of interest, no gross deficits in Anne's visual fields could be appreciated—that is, there were no specific areas in either her central or peripheral vision that were substantially worse than the others. Anne's ophthalmologist felt that her presentation was most consistent with a cataracts—a problem with the lens of the eye that is relatively common in older patients. Anne agreed to the standard surgical treatment for cataracts. After the procedure, however, both she and her doctor were surprised that her visual symptoms had not improved.

Six months later, Anne's condition had grown considerably worse. She had begun to suffer from headaches. Her issues with eyesight had continued to worsen. Her short-term memory loss was now severe. Around this time, Anne's ophthalmologist sent her to a second doctor specializing in neuro-ophthalmology. The neuro-ophthalmologist was very troubled to hear of Anne's symptoms and ordered magnetic resonance imaging (MRI) of her brain. The MRI revealed a large tumor filling the third ventricle—a cavity immediately behind the optic chiasm and resting in between the hypothalamic centers (Figure 9.1). The tumor was associated with extensive inflammation that was almost certainly the cause of Anne's visual symptoms and memory loss.

After the discovery of the tumor, Anne's physician referred her to Dr. Jonathan Forbes, a neurosurgeon specializing in treatment of cranial tumors. Dr. Forbes explained the location of the tumor in relation

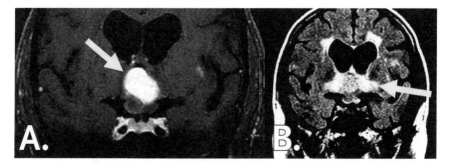

FIGURE 9.1 Pre-operative MRI. MRI (A) demonstrates a chordoid glioma (yellow arrow) occupying the confines of the third ventricle that appears bright after being injected with contrast. The underlying optic nerves and chiasm are swollen and inflamed. MRI (B) shows extensive tissue damage associated with the mass (yellow arrow) that appears as a bright signal.

to important surrounding structures. He described how the extensive tumor-associated inflammation in the adjacent hypothalamus and optic tracts was likely responsible for Anne's symptoms. Dr. Forbes recommended an initial ventriculoscopic biopsy to determine the type of tumor and whether any non-surgical options for treatment might exist. Anne consented for this biopsy, which was performed without complication. The tumor was identified by the neuropathology team as a chordoid glioma. At a brain tumor conference, the risks of conservative management were weighed against the risks of surgical resection. In the setting of progressive deterioration in vision and memory linked to tumor-associated inflammation, surgical resection was recommended.[5] Anne discussed the plan of care with Dr. Forbes and agreed to proceed with definitive resection of the tumor.

A minimally invasive, right trans-ventricular, trans-choroidal fissure approach was selected for definitive treatment. In the procedure, Dr. Forbes advanced a small tubular retractor into the ventricular system. The choroidal fissure, or the natural cleft between the fornix and thalamus, was gently opened—providing access to the third ventricle. Under high magnification, the tumor was meticulously removed. Following surgery, MRI demonstrated appropriate resection of the tumor with complete resolution

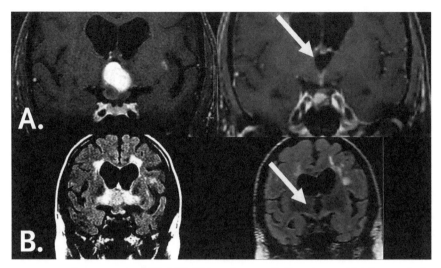

FIGURE 9.2   Post-operative MRI. MRI (A) imaging pre- (left) and post- (right) operatively. The yellow arrow points to the third ventricle after the brightly appearing tumor was removed. The optic apparatus, seen below the third ventricle, has returned to normal size following tumor removal. MRI (B) shows significant improvement in the tissue damage associated with the tumor seen by the bright white signal pre- (left) and post- (right) operatively. The yellow arrow highlights the lack of inflammation in this region after the tumor excision.

of tumor-associated inflammation in the hypothalamus and optic tracts (Figure 9.2). The physical therapy team helped Anne speed through her recovery. Her visual symptoms had improved within a few days. Anne had noted marked improvement in short-term memory only a few weeks following the surgery. Three months after the surgery, Anne had regained her old form at Sudoku and resumed many of her old hobbies. In the months ahead, Anne would recover the high quality of life she enjoyed prior to the tumor and even find time to crochet an incredible doll for Dr. Forbes and the neurosurgery team.

ENDNOTES

1. S. Chibbaro et al., "Neuroendoscopic management of posterior third ventricle and pineal region tumors: Technique, limitation, and possible complication avoidance," *Neurosurgical Review* 35, no. 3 (2012): 331-340, https://doi.org/10.1007/s10143 -011-0370-1.
2. Syed I. Ahmed et al., "Third Ventricular Tumors: A Comprehensive Literature Review," *Cureus* 10, no. 10 (October 2018): e3417, https://doi.org/10.7759/cureus.3417
3. Yasuo Sugita et al., "The tumor of the third ventricle," *Neuropathology* 30 (2010): 97-100, https://doi.org/10.1111/j.1440-1789.2009.01057.x
4. D. J. Vanhauwaert et al., "Chordoid glioma of the third ventricle," *Acta Neurochirurgica* 150, no. 11 (2008): 1183-1191, https://doi.org/10.1007/s00701-008-0014-6.
5. Gregorio Zlotnik and Aaron Vansintjan, "Memory: An Extended Definition," *Frontiers in Psychology* 10 (November 2019): 2523. https://doi.org/10.3389/fpsyg .2019.02523.

REFERENCES

Ahmed, Syed I., Gohar Javed, Altaf Ali Laghari, Syeda Beenish Bareeqa, Kashif Aziz, Mehreen Khan, Syeda Sana Samar, Raja Azhar Humera, Alizay Rashid Khan, Muhammad Osama Farooqui, Amir Shahbaz. "Third Ventricular Tumors: A Comprehensive Literature Review." *Cureus* 10, no. 10 (October 2018): e3417, https://doi .org/10.7759/cureus.3417

Kuramoto, Kenji Nakayama. "The tumor of the third ventricle." *Neuropathology* 30 (2010): 97-100, https://doi.org/10.1111/j.1440-1789.2009.01057.x

Sugita, Yasuo, Koichi Ohshima, Minoru Shigemori, Masahiro Arakawa, Teruaki Chibbaro, S., F. Di Rocco, O. Makiese, A. Reiss, P. Poczos, G. Mirone, F. Servadei, B. George, P. Crafa, M. Polivka, A. Romano. "Neuroendoscopic management of posterior third ventricle and pineal region tumors: Technique, limitation, and possible complication avoidance." *Neurosurgical Review* 35, no. 3 (2012): 331-340, https://doi .org/10.1007/s10143-011-0370-1.

Vanhauwaert, D.J., F Clement, J Van Dorpe, M J Deruytter. "Chordoid glioma of the third ventricle." *Acta Neurochirurgica* 150, no. 11 (2008): 1183-1191, https://doi .org/10.1007/s00701-008-0014-6.

Zlotnik, Gregorio and Aaron Vansintjan. "Memory: An Extended Definition," Frontiers in Psychology 10 (November 2019): 2523. https://doi.org/10.3389/fpsyg.2019.02523.

COMPENDIUM

RICHARD BECKER, MD, MED, FAHA

JAMIE DENLINGER, RN, BSN

MELISSA ERICKSON, MD

ALBERTO ESPAY, MD, MSC, FAAN

JONATHAN A. FORBES, MD

MLADEN GOLUBIC, MD, PHD

MARCIA KAPLAN, MD

MICHELLE KIRSCHNER, MSN, RN, ACNP, APRN-BC

ABIGAIL KOEHLER, BS

HEATHER RAVVIN MCKEE, MD

YEHUDIT ROTHMAN, PA-C

ALI J. ZARRABI, MD

SOMA SENGUPTA, MD, PHD, FRCP

KYLE WANG, MD

The following compendium is designed to share information and resources for patients, their loved ones, and/or caregivers who have received a new brain tumor diagnosis or have previously been diagnosed with brain tumors. Some of the resources listed, including contact information referenced, are specifically available at the University of Cincinnati Medical Center/UC Health. If you are not located in the Greater Cincinnati area, please reach out to your preferred healthcare provider to inquire whether similar resources are available in your area.

BRAIN-TUMOR RELATED EPILEPSY

Seizures are the most common symptom caused by brain tumors.[1] The overall frequency of seizures accompanying brain tumors ranges from 35%

to 70%.[2] Epilepsy in patients with brain tumors is considered the most significant risk factor for long-term disability.[3] Epilepsy is defined as a patient having two or more seizures, or one seizure in a patient whose abnormal magnetic resonance imaging (MRI) or electroencephalography (EEG) indicates an increased risk for future seizures.[4] Patients with a brain tumor and seizures meet the criteria for a diagnosis of epilepsy, and hence treatment for their epilepsy is warranted.[5] There is not, however, any strong evidence that anti-seizure medication (ASM) prescribed to patients with brain tumors but no history of seizures is an effective treatment, so the decision to utilize that kind of medication should be guided by an assessment of individual risk factors and careful discussion with a neurologist.[6] It is recommended to see a neurologist after a seizure occurs, as patients with brain tumor-related epilepsy present a complex therapeutic profile and require a unique and multidisciplinary approach. It is not unusual to have some amount of trial and error with anti-seizure medications, as there is not any one medication indicated for a particular brain tumor, and patients may require more than one medication for optimal seizure control. Importantly, full compliance with medication is essential.

Brain tumor-related epilepsy falls into the focal epilepsy category, given that a localized abnormality in the brain is the cause of the seizures. This allows for a broad range of treatment options for patients with brain tumor-related epilepsy, which includes broad-spectrum anti-seizure medications (ASMs) and ASMs used for focal epilepsy only. When deciding on a treatment option, it is critical to consider other medications, existing medical conditions, and potential side effects.[7] ASMs that are often considered first when treating brain tumor-related epilepsy are ones with the fewest drug interactions, potential side effects, require minimal laboratory follow up, and are generic, so approval is easily obtainable, such as levetiracetam and lamotrigine. Levetiracetam can have a therapeutic effect that is relatively immediate, whereas lamotrigine requires an initial seven-week gradual dose increase to avoid a rash as a possible side effect, which limits immediate use. Lamotrigine, overall, is well-tolerated and typically the most highly recommended anti-seizure medication in older adults (>55 years).[8]

Levetiracetam is also typically well-tolerated, but potential side effects can include negative effects on mood, fatigue, and rarely could cause cytopenia (low blood cell count). Oxcarbazepine is another medication option, but it carries the possible side effect of hyponatremia (low sodium), particularly in older patients. Second-line brand name options include lacosamide, brivaracetam, or other broad-spectrum medications including valproic acid, zonisamide, or topiramate. Some medications may require cardiac screening with an electrocardiogram (EKG). Recommendations include the avoidance of an older category of ASMs that have stronger effects on drug metabolism and can interfere with anti-tumoral medications.[9] The main ASMs in this category are phenytoin, carbamazepine, phenobarbital, and primidone.[10] An epilepsy specialist would be able to provide the highest trained care for these patients and tailor their medication choice according to individual patient needs. Successful treatment is complete seizure freedom. Additional resources and information are available on the Epilepsy Foundation's website: www.epilepsy.com.

DEPRESSION FOLLOWING BRAIN TUMOR DIAGNOSIS

Any patient facing a brain tumor diagnosis can experience distress. Depression and anxiety are highly prevalent even among members of the general population who have no related underlying medical conditions. To develop a clearer understanding of the phenomena linking brain tumors, depression, and anxiety, patients should be asked if they had mood and anxiety symptoms that developed before a brain tumor diagnosis or afterward as a result of their diagnosis. Is there biologically mediated change in mood and anxiety-regulating mechanisms in patients with brain tumors, and if so, what mechanisms might cause such symptoms? Did these symptoms develop before the brain tumor was large enough to cause symptoms, or only after the tumor was discovered? And finally, if patients with brain tumors have significant mood changes and anxiety symptoms, how do we best treat them?

It has been noted that depressive symptoms in patients with primary brain tumors are independently associated with reduced quality of life and survival time.[11] Researchers suggest that underlying inflammatory activation modulated through proinflammatory cytokines might cause depression as they promote tumor growth and metastasis. Additionally, they suggest that the tumor microenvironment might render treatment for depression less effective. One study reported on a sample of 89 patients with brain tumors which showed that 28% of those patients met the criteria for major depression. Major depression was predicted by the location of the tumor in the frontal lobe, combined with sadness, lack of motivation, and family psychiatric history.[12] Researchers attempted a meta-analysis of the course of patients with primary brain tumors but found obstacles to identifying these patients due to exclusion criteria such as cognitive impairment.[13] Of the small sample they identified, existential distress was correlated with significant depression, anxiety, and overall worse quality of life. Depression was studied across a wide range of neurological conditions including tumors of the brain and spine in over 4,000 patients and researchers found that the highest prevalence of depression (over 30% of the sample) occurred in those with traumatic brain injury (TBI) and brain tumors.[14] Another study looked at 159 patients undergoing craniotomy for tumor resection and found that 48% reported high levels of distress and nearly seven sources of cancer-related distress.[15]

In a retrospective chart review of 301 deceased patients with primary or metastatic brain tumors, Appleby et al. found that depression was the most common premorbid psychiatric symptom, followed by substance abuse and anxiety.[16] Comorbid depression developed in 15% and anxiety developed in 12% of their sample. Depression was as likely to be reported in male and female subjects, while anxiety was 3 times more likely to develop in female subjects. 34 depressed subjects were prescribed antidepressant medications and only 12 met with a psychiatrist at some point during their illness. Premorbid depression and anxiety were highly predictive of worse symptoms after diagnosis. Their findings make clear a significant underestimation and under-reporting of mood and anxiety symptoms in brain tumor patients, as well as a lack of psychiatric assessment for many of these patients.

There are case reports of individuals with psychiatric illness in whom brain tumors are later discovered.[17] These anecdotal reports do prove a coorelation between mood and anxiety problems, which are common, with brain tumor development nor do they suggest that brain imaging is recommended for depressed and anxious patients without focal neurological symptoms. On the other hand, primary care physicians and psychiatrists must maintain a high degree of suspicion if patients develop mood or anxiety symptoms with abrupt or late-onset when there are concurrent neurologic focal signs.

Once diagnosed, patients with brain tumors should be monitored for their level of distress, capacity to sleep, eat, concentrate, and maintain meaningful activities and relationships.[18] Married patients may be better protected from distress and have reported only half as much anxiety as single patients.[19] Supportive services should be offered early in the process of treatment, whether those embedded in oncology treatment centers or through community-supported agencies in many communities that offer individual and group psychotherapy and psychoeducation both for the patient and their families. Often general supportive treatment approaches are adequate for relief. Eye movement desensitization and reprocessing (EMDR) treatment, originally developed as a treatment for posttraumatic stress disorder (PTSD), was found to be statistically significant over standard medical care for improving depression, anxiety, and anger in patients with glioblastoma multiforme.[20] When psychological symptoms are severe, psychiatric evaluation is appropriate, but where this is not available, primary care physicians or oncologists should consider prescribing serotonergic antidepressants.[21] For patients with more troubling symptoms, including insomnia and nausea, second-generation antipsychotics 20-50 mg of quetiapine and 2.5-5 mg of olanzapine taken at bedtime can provide significant relief.

RESOURCES FOLLOWING DIAGNOSIS

NURSE NAVIGATION

Many patients find themselves overwhelmed following a brain tumor diagnosis. It may be challenging to keep track of all the information provided during appointments, including the timeline of the treatment plan itself, while simultaneously juggling the stress of their new diagnosis. This is where a nurse navigator steps in. The main role of nurse navigation for brain tumor patients, or any other cancer type, is to ensure that the often disparate parts of the overall treatment team/plan are interconnected to ensure timely, complete, and quality care. The figure below shows a flow-chart of a typical treatment plan for newly diagnosed brain tumor patients.

There are many aspects to a patient's treatment plan. The plan often begins with an initial visit to a neurosurgeon. It is at this point that nurse navigation can make a stressful situation somewhat less stressful. A comprehensive approach to patient care includes a dedicated team member contacting the patient and/or their family after the initial appointments to follow-up on comprehension of the diagnosis and discussion of possible

An MRI is done with and without contrast suggestive of a brain tumor

A neurosurgeon will remove as much of the tumor as safely possible

If complete resection of the tumor is achieved and the pathology is consistent with a GBM, about four weeks of healing time with additional treatment is estimated

The patient sees radiation oncology for radiation planning and neuro-oncology for chemotherapy management and to discuss possible clinical trials.

surgical interventions. Establishing a rapport with a team member at this stage builds trust and confidence in the health care system. A nurse navigator meets with patients and their families again after surgery to ensure that these patients are seeing the correct providers and are connected with resources to help them cope with the physical and emotional consequences of the tumor, and possibly, the surgery.

Nurse navigation also plays an essential role in post-treatment and survivorship. As the patient progresses beyond the active treatment stage, it is possible to lose these patients to follow-up. The nurse navigator is the member of the treatment team that reaches out to provide support and keep the patient in touch with the healthcare system.[22]

PRIMARY CARE

At the University of Cincinnati Medical Center (UCMC), a large percentage of cancer patients either did not have a primary care physician or felt that their primary care physicians were not well-versed in the long-term effects of their cancer treatment. Utilizing a model proposed by Dr. Larissa Nekhlyudov of the Brigham and Women's Hospital, UCMC created an oncology primary care clinic that is embedded in the institution's cancer center.[23] The goal of the clinic is to provide comprehensive primary care for patients with a history of cancer. It is staffed by a family medicine physician with additional training and experience in cancer survivorship. The proximity to treatment specialists has helped facilitate communication, allowing for more coordinated care, and it has also helped prevent potential delays in treatment by monitoring such conditions as severe hyperglycemia and elevated blood pressure. Additionally, this hospital-based model allows for improved mental health services, including access to social workers and medication management for anxiety and depression, which are diagnoses that primary care physicians are well-suited to treat.

SURVIVORSHIP CARE

Survivorship care focuses on meeting the comprehensive needs of patients who have been diagnosed with tumors. Most often, it centers on cancer patients who have malignant tumors. However, for those with brain tumors, survivorship care can also include benign (non-cancerous) tumors along with malignant tumors. In fact, patients with a benign brain tumor may often have access to some of the same survivorship services as those living with a malignant brain tumor. This is because benign and malignant brain tumors impact a person's overall health in similar ways. For this reason, the National Cancer Registry requires hospitals to track benign brain tumor patients together with their cancer patients.

According to the National Cancer Institute's Office of Cancer Survivorship, "zn individual is considered a cancer survivor from the time of diagnosis, through the balance of his or her life. There are many types of *survivors*, including those living with cancer and those free of cancer."[24] Survivorship care moves beyond the treatment of the tumor itself, focusing instead on the mental, emotional, physical, and spiritual impact on the individual and the caregiver.

Historically, survivorship services were focused on the delivery of a "survivorship care plan" document at the end of active treatment. Over time, survivorship care has become more collaborative and now emphasizes ongoing supportive services for patients. As part of this shift, the survivorship world is now exploring the needs of patients during different phases of treatment such as receiving therapy with curative intent for new diagnoses, post active treatment (on or off maintenance therapy), or living with cancer as a chronic condition.[25] The expansion of survivorship care has created diversity in the types and availability of care that are organized. Large academic centers often lead this process through survivorship research and innovative programs. At the University of Cincinnati Medical Center (UCMC), the Neuro-Oncology and Survivorship programs have collaborated to create a Brain Tumor Survivorship Clinic. The goal of this clinic is to establish a relationship early on with the patient and caregiver to complete a comprehensive intake assessment and administer baseline cognitive testing, when appropriate.

Brain tumors can affect almost any region of the brain. Many tumors can then disrupt networks associated with cognitive function. As such, tumors can directly affect patients' ability to communicate, socialize, interact, and even carry out daily activities. Some of the difficulties are hard to measure during a clinic visit and may require the evaluation of a neuropsychologist to determine the areas affected including visuospatial orientation, executive function, naming, memory, attention, or language.[26] For this reason, the Neuro-Oncology clinic uses the National Institute of Health (NIH) Toolbox Cognition Battery (Age 12+) and the Consortium to Establish a Registry for Alzheimer's Disease (CERAD) batteries for cognitive testing. These batteries provide explicit details on which aspects of cognition are impaired. The data collected from patients is then interpreted by a neurocognition specialist.

Survivorship care for this population is focused on addressing the impact of the tumor on their quality of life and potential interventions.[27] The patient is considered a partner in the process, and self-management is reinforced through the provision of resources for their journey. Overall wellness is promoted through education on the benefits of exercise, optimal nutrition, and mindfulness meditation. The clinic has been structured to highlight the specific effects of a brain tumor and its impact. For example, cognition is supported by determining potential areas of optimization including exploring the status of sleep, pain, and psychosocial inputs. Individuals are followed by the survivorship care team through telehealth and/or in-person visits to allow for the continued customization of recommendations.

Brain tumor patients and their caregivers must be aware that there may be helpful services and programs available through survivorship care. Health care providers within the survivorship program may have supportive care visits available, in which a global assessment of needs can be conducted, and then individuals can be connected to these services. The benefit of working with a survivorship team is that they are often familiar with the specific needs of the brain tumor population and can efficiently direct patients to the most appropriate services. If a health care system does not have a structured survivorship program, there may be resources through a regional academic center.

NAUSEA DURING BRAIN TUMOR TREATMENT

While undergoing treatment of a brain tumor, many patients will experience nausea as an unwelcomed side effect. A neuro-oncologist will typically prescribe an anti-nausea medication to take prior to the beginning of chemotherapy. Because there are many different classes and types of anti-nausea medications, it is important to work with a neuro-oncologist to find the right regimen. Even more important than the type of anti-nausea medication is the timing of the medication. It is much harder to control nausea once a patient is already feeling symptomatic. It is better to pre-empt nausea by taking anti-nausea medication before receiving chemotherapy.[28] If a patient typically feels nauseous throughout their treatment, they should have one medication that is taken every 6-8 hours regardless of being symptomatic, as well as a second medication to take as needed for breakthrough nausea.

In addition to medications and medical management, there are also lifestyle changes and alternative treatments that may help with nausea. Eating bland, easy to digest foods and avoiding spicy, sweet, or fatty foods may help control nausea.[29] Staying away from strong smells, eating cold or room temperature foods, and staying well hydrated can also help to keep nausea under control.[30] Some alternative treatments may include peppermint tea or essential oils, ginger tea, real ginger ale, or ginger candies.[31] Acupuncture, as well as acupressure bands, have been helpful for some people.[32] If you are interested, talk with your doctor about getting a referral for acupuncture services at UC Health.

INTEGRATIVE MEDICINE FOR PATIENTS WITH BRAIN TUMORS

Thirty to eighty percent of patients diagnosed with cancer, including brain tumors, often use therapeutic modalities of integrative medicine. Their desire to actively contribute to the treatment of their disease and relieve symptoms associated with modern medical and surgical therapies seems to be the driving motivation.

The field of integrative medicine encompasses a spectrum of complementary evidence-based cancer care practices, alongside conventional cancer therapies. It combines the best of modern molecular medicine with known holistic therapies. The dedication to scientific research and evidence-based practice by practitioners of integrative medicine stands in sharp contrast to proponents of a variety of alternative treatments based on unsubstantiated claims that cancer can be cured exclusively through alternative therapies instead of conventional cancer treatments.

Integrative medicine includes, among other things, lifestyle modifications, mind-body and movement practices, and different modalities from traditional medical systems such as acupuncture and natural products (herbs, vitamins, minerals, and probiotics). The focus of these integrative therapies is to engage patients with their self-care, include their families as active participants throughout treatment and survivorship, facilitate positive behavior changes, help manage cancer-related symptoms, and improve quality of life.

Health challenges are frequently encountered by patients affected by brain tumors, such as fatigue, pain, sleep difficulties, neuropathy, and anxiety. These challenges can often be alleviated by therapeutic modalities of integrative medicine. At the University of Cincinnati Center for Integrative Health and Wellness, we use a spectrum of therapies for these and other symptoms as recommended by the leading national professional cancer organizations. Those therapies include acupuncture, massage therapy, yoga, Tai Chi, music/art therapy, mindfulness meditation, and lifestyle medicine consultation with physicians.

Helping cancer patients cultivate health-promoting lifestyle habits is the foundation of current recommendations by the American Cancer Society, the American Institute for Cancer Research, and other organizations for expanding cancer treatment to include the promotion of overall long-term health. The inclusion of experts in nutrition, exercise science, and behavioral change has been shown to have a beneficial impact on a wide range of health outcomes. For example, adherence to a predominantly plant-based eating pattern that is rich in vegetables, whole grains, legumes, and fruits, with minimal consumption of processed foods, sugars, alcohol, and red and processed meats is considered a cornerstone of care for cancer survivors. Dietary patterns that reduce inflammation, such as the

Mediterranean diet and other plant-based diets, may also reduce fatigue.

The National Comprehensive Cancer Network Guidelines recommend the use of acupuncture for pain, fatigue, nausea, and vomiting. Massage therapy has been shown to reduce cancer-related fatigue, pain, psychological stress, and to improve mood. Regular practice of mindfulness-based techniques can lead to decreased fatigue, depression, anxiety, chronic stress, and pain, to improved sleep and quality of life in general. It is also critical in the development and maintenance of health-promoting lifestyle habits and the avoidance of risky behaviors, such as smoking and alcohol consumption.

Compelling evidence supports cancer patients' use of meditative movement practices such as Tai Chi and yoga for improving the quality of emotional health, sleep, balance, and for reducing the risk of falls. Considering the well-demonstrated benefits of physical activity for cancer survivors (increased vigor and vitality, better sleep, improved quality of life, cardiorespiratory fitness, decreased depression, anxiety, and fatigue), yoga and/or Tai Chi practice could be particularly helpful for patients who are weak and too fatigued to engage safely in physical activity. Although continuous, rigorously designed research on integrative therapies and self-care practices is necessary, the currently available knowledge forms a solid basis for sorely needed explorations on the best ways to widely implement such therapies in everyday clinical practice in a sustainable and equitable manner.[33]

ADDRESSING THE SYMPTOMS: PALLIATIVE CARE

Palliative care, also known as supportive care, is both an approach to care and a medical subspecialty that addresses the symptoms and stress of a serious illness, such as brain tumors. It is appropriate at any age or any stage in a serious illness and is based on the needs of the patient rather than the patient's prognosis.[34] More specifically, palliative care assesses and addresses physical, intellectual, social, emotional, and spiritual needs by anticipating, preventing, and alleviating suffering throughout the continuum of an individual's illness.[35] Palliative care is provided by a specially trained interdisciplinary team of doctors, nurses, and other specialists, such as social workers and chaplains, who work with the patient's other doctors, specifically neurologists and oncologists, to provide an extra layer of support.[36] Over two decades of evidence supports the use of palliative care across care settings, from the hospital to the clinic, to improve the quality of life of seriously ill patients and their families.[37] Furthermore, emerging evidence suggests that when palliative care is provided in the outpatient setting to patients with advanced cancers, the patient's prognosis may also improve.[38]

Patients with brain tumors can experience symptoms that can impact their quality of life including headaches, insomnia, fatigue, cachexia, altered mental status, and cognitive impairment.[39] Furthermore, patients may experience isolation, anxiety, depression, demoralization, and existential distress, particularly as some approach the end of life.[40] Specialists in palliative care can identify constellations of physical symptoms and emotional distress and tailor treatment plans for individual patients with brain tumors. Furthermore, teams can support patients' loved ones and coordinate care with other healthcare professionals. The landscape of palliative care's scope of practice is not yet standardized, and thus both the scope and practice of palliative care are variable across the United States.[41] For this reason, patients and family members should ask their healthcare providers about how to access palliative care services and what services are specifically offered when confronting a serious illness such as a brain tumor.

Depending on the state in the US, guidelines regarding marijuana use differ. It is useful in brain tumor patients and has been said to improve, mood, appetite, and sleep. There is a pilot clinical trial to suggest that (Δ9) tetrahydrocannabinol (THC) might be useful in glioma patients.[42] In many instances, marijuana palliates brain tumor patient symptoms more than opioids with fewer side effects. A reputable marijuana pharmacy should be used if the neuro-oncologist is not permitted to prescribe it in a given healthcare system.

HEART CONDITIONS

A relationship between brain tumors and heart conditions can take several forms. First, health conditions like high blood pressure, high cholesterol, and diabetes, or risky behaviors such as smoking contribute to the hardening of the arteries, also referred to as atherosclerosis. They can also lead to a heart attack, which might require a stent or bypass surgery, or a stroke, which can cause difficulty with speaking, walking, and coordination and balance, or a weakened heart muscle.[43] Second, brain tumors, particularly large tumors associated with swelling in the brain itself, cause high blood pressure and either a slow or irregular heart rhythm. Third, tumors within specific parts of the brain can alter the heart and circulation's abilities to regulate heart rate and blood pressure in response to changes in posture (lying, sitting, or standing) or the environment (heat, humidity, and cold conditions). As a result, the heart can beat very fast (>100 beats per minute) when standing, or the blood pressure can either increase when lying down or suddenly drop when sitting, standing, or walking. Symptoms can develop such as heart racing, palpitations, sweating, worsening headaches, dizziness, or loss of consciousness.[44] Finally, some but not all cancer-related treatments, such as chemotherapy or immunotherapy, have side effects that can cause cardiomyopathy, an increase or decrease in blood pressure, alterations in heart rate or rhythm, or can heighten the blood's ability to form blood clots. The latter is the proximate cause of heart attack, stroke, deep vein thrombosis, and pulmonary embolism.[45]

The most common signs or symptoms of a heart condition are chest pain, shortness of breath, rapidly progressive fatigue or impaired stamina, swelling of the legs, rapid weight gain, dizziness, lightheadedness or passing out with a change in posture, heart racing or fluttering, and worsening headache when lying down.

A heart specialist or cardiologist is often a member of the brain tumor team. She or he will perform an assessment by reviewing past medical history of heart conditions, risk factors for heart disease, and planned treatment. A thorough physical examination, electrocardiogram (EKG), and echocardiogram are common tests performed in this assessment. Other tests recommended by a heart specialist, often referred to as a cardio-oncologist, may include an MRI of the heart, Holter monitor (tape recording of the hearts rhythm), and a coronary computerized tomography (CT) angio-gram to evaluate for narrowing of one or more blood vessels providing blood and oxygen to the heart.

THE BASICS OF NAVIGATING CLINICAL TRIALS

It is common for brain tumor patients to join clinical trials, especially those diagnosed with glioblastoma multiforme (GBM). Clinical trials, though considered experimental, offer unique treatments for patients, and contrib-ute to ongoing research investigating different treatments. Clinical trials typically have four steps, each focusing heavily on background research and data review to evaluate safety and effectiveness. The following flow chart diagram shows the different phases of a typical clinical trial, and what each step entails for researchers and research subjects.

The World Health Organization (WHO) is a prominent United Nations health agency that serves to promote global health. The WHO sets staging/grading requirements and identifies molecular or histological markers of brain tumors that can be used to further classify them. These classifications are often heavily considered when determining the course of treatment, as some molecular characteristics may be targetable by drugs or other anti-cancer therapies. 2021 WHO guidelines for brain tumors are a further reference, and many centers perform Caris or Foundation One sequenc-ing of more aggressive brain tumors to help guide future therapy options. The discussion of molecular signatures is not the purpose of this book. Recently, the 5th edition of the World Health Organization Classification of Tumors of the Central Nervous System was released, where the WHO amended their guidelines to update the classifications of brain tumors.[46] WHO guidelines are extremely relevant for GBM clinical trials because these trials are based on these guidelines. Patients or their caregivers can explore available clinical trials on www.clinicaltrials.gov.

Clinicaltrials.gov is a database of all the clinical trials around the world. Patients can look up studies based on their condition/disease, location, or other parameters such as the investigational device/drug or name of the investigator. Advanced criteria that may narrow the search include the type

PHASE 0 — Micro-dosing studies; speeds up drug/immunotherapy development

PHASE 1 — Testing a drug/immunotherapy in healthy volunteers; evaluates the safety of a study drug

PHASE 2 — Testing a drug/immunotherapy in patient population; evaluates drug/immunotherapy safety and efficacy

PHASE 3 — Usually requires many patients; evaluates how well the new agent performs compared to a readily available drug

or phase of the study, stage of recruitment, eligibility criteria, type of study intervention, or funding entity. Study-specific criteria such as the name of the researcher, study title, or identification numbers can also be searched. It is important to double check that the search contains the condition or disease of interest and the correct location (country, state, and/or city), otherwise, the search will include clinical trials that are unavailable in your area.

The status of the clinical trial is displayed next to the study title and states whether patients can join the study. A green "Recruiting" status means that the study is currently open, and patients may join. A green "Not yet recruiting" status means that the study may soon be opening and looking for patients to join. The conditions of research interest, the type of intervention being studied, and the location where the study is being conducted are also listed on the search page. Additional information, including a description of the research and who to contact about participation, can be found by clicking on the title of the study.

OVERVIEW OF RADIATION THERAPY FOR BRAIN TUMORS

Radiation is used for many types of brain tumors, sometimes with surgery and chemotherapy, and works by damaging DNA and affecting tumor cell division. Radiation is usually delivered with photons, which are x-rays. There are two different types of radiation therapy: intensity modulated radiation therapy (IMRT) that consists of ~15-30 low dose treatments and stereotactic radiosurgery (SRS) that consists of ~1-5 high-dose treatments. Both IMRT and SRS use many radiation beams from multiple directions that all focus on the target, so that the radiation dose to the tumor is maximized and the dose to surrounding organs minimized. Radiation can also be delivered with proton particles, which use fewer beams and can further lower the radiation dose to parts of the brain and other organs not near the tumor.[47] IMRT or proton radiation are usually recommended for gliomas and large tumors, whereas SRS is usually recommended for brain metastases or small, benign tumors.

The first step is a radiation planning scan (or simulation CT), usually one to two weeks before starting treatment. For this procedure, the patient is placed flat on a table in the treatment position and a see-through mask is used to immobilize the patient's head. Medications can be used to help patients who are claustrophobic or anxious about the mask. The radiation oncologist will then use the planning scan and other scans, such as an MRI, to design the radiation plan. Before each treatment, a quick scan is performed to make sure everything lines up to the planning scan accurately. The actual treatment itself may last anywhere from five to thirty minutes and does not hurt. The body is better at repairing the effects of radiation than of tumors, but radiation can cause side effects during or within a few weeks or months after treatment. Depending on the location and tumor size, these side effects can include fatigue, nausea, headaches from brain swelling, hair loss, and neurocognitive disturbances.[48] With higher radiation doses, swelling can appear long after radiation and even be confused with tumor. For patients with severe symptoms due to swelling, steroid medications, such as dexamethasone, are often used. Every patient and tumor are different, but the radiation oncologist will always try to minimize the risk of side effects through careful treatment planning.

ENDNOTES

1. Marta Maschio et al., "Weight of Epilepsy in Brain Tumor Patients," *Journal of Neuro-Oncology* 118, no. 2 (May 2014): 385-393. https://doi.org/10.1007/s11060-014 -1449-7.

2. M.J. Glantz et al., "Practice Parameter: Anticonvulsant Prophylaxis in Patients with Newly Diagnosed Brain Tumors. Report of the Quality Standards Subcommittee of the American Academy of Neurology," *Neurology* 54, no. 10 (May 2000): 1886–93. https://doi.org/10.1212/wnl.54.10.1886; Charles Vecht and Erik B. Wilms, "Seizures in Low- and High-Grade Gliomas: Current Management and Future Outlook," *Expert Review of Anticancer Therapy* 10, no. 5 (May 2010): 663–69. https://doi .org/10.1586/era.10.48.

3. Marta Maschio et al., "Weight of Epilepsy in Brain Tumor Patients," 385-393; M. Maschio et al., "Antiepileptics in Brain Metastases: Safety, Efficacy and Impact on Life Expectancy," *Journal of Neuro-Oncology* 98 (2009): 109–16. https://doi.org /10.1007/s11060-009-0069-0.

4. Robert Fisher et al., "ILAE Official Report: A Practical Clinical Definition of Epilepsy," *Epilepsia* 55, no. 4 (April 2014): 475–82. https://doi.org/10.1111/epi.12550.

5. M.J. Glantz et al., "Practice Parameter: Anticonvulsant Prophylaxis in Patients with Newly Diagnosed Brain Tumors. Report of the Quality Standards Subcommittee of the American Academy of Neurology," 1886-93: Marta Maschio et al., "Management of Epilepsy in Brain Tumors," *Neurological Sciences* 40, no. 10 (October 2019): 2217–34. https://doi.org/10.1007/s10072-019-04025-9; Allan Krumholz et al., "Evidence-Based Guideline: Management of an Unprovoked First Seizure in Adults: Report of the Guideline Development Subcommittee of the American Academy of Neurology and the American Epilepsy Society," *Neurology* 84, no. 16 (April 2015): 1705–13. https://doi.org/10.1212/WNL.0000000000001487; Anne T. Berg, "Risk of Recurrence after a First Unprovoked Seizure," *Epilepsia* 49 (2008): 13–18. https://doi.org/10.1111/j.1528-1167.2008.01444.x; J.F. Annegers et al., "Risk of Recurrence after an Initial Unprovoked Seizure," *Epilepsia* 27, no. 1 (February 1986): 43–50. https://doi.org/10.1111/j.1528-1157.1986.tb03499.x; P. Jallon, P. Loiseau, J. and Loiseau, "Newly Diagnosed Unprovoked Epileptic Seizures: Presentation at Diagnosis in CAROLE Study. Coordination Active Du Réseau Observatoire Longitudinal de l'Epilepsie," *Epilepsia* 42, no. 4 (April 2001): 464–75. https://doi.org /10.1046/j.1528-1157.2001.31400.x.

6. M.J. Glantz et al., "Practice Parameter: Anticonvulsant Prophylaxis in Patients with Newly Diagnosed Brain Tumors. Report of the Quality Standards Subcommittee of the American Academy of Neurology," *Neurology* 54, no. 10 (May 2000): 1883-1893. https://doi.org/10.1212/wnl.54.10.1886. Elaine Wyllie, "Encephalopathic Generalized Epilepsy and Lennox-Gastaut Syndrome," in *Wyllie's Treatment of Epilepsy: Principles and Practice*, 6th edition (Philadelphia, PA: Wolters Kluwer, 2015),

272–83; I.W. Tremont-Lukats, et al. "Antiepileptic Drugs for Preventing Seizures in People with Brain Tumors," *Cochrane Database System Review* no. 2 (April 2008): CD004424. https://doi.org/10.1002/14651858.CD004424.pub2.

7. Marta Maschio et al., "Management of Epilepsy in Brain Tumors," 2217–34.

8. Hilba Arif et al., "Comparative Effectiveness of 10 Antiepileptic Drugs in Older Adults with Epilepsy," *Archives of Neurology* 67, no. 4 (April 2010): 408–15. https://doi.org/10.1001/archneurol.2010.49.

9. Marta Maschio et al., "Management of Epilepsy in Brain Tumors," 2217–34.

10. Emilio Perucca, "Clinically Relevant Drug Interactions with Antiepileptic Drugs," *British Journal of Clinical Pharmacology* 61, no. 3 (March 2006): 246–55. https://doi.org/10.1111/j.1365-2125.2005.02529.x.

11. Angela Starkweather et al., "A Biobehavioral Perspective on Depressive Symptoms in Patients with Cerebral Astrocytomas," *Journal of Neuroscience Nursing* 43, no. 1 (2011): 17–28. https://doi.org/10.1097/jnn.0b013e3182029859.

12. David Wellisch et al., "Predicting Major Depression in Brain Tumor Patients," *Psycho-Oncology* 11, no. 3 (2002): 230–38. https://doi.org/10.1002/pon.562.

13. Ashlee Loughan et al., "Fear of Cancer Recurrence and Death Anxiety: Unaddressed Concerns for Adult Neuro-Oncology Patients," *Journal of Clinical Psychology in Medical Settings* 28, no. 1 (2021): 16–30. https://doi.org/10.1007/s10880-019-09690-8.

14. Andrew Bulloch et al., "Depression—a Common Disorder across Broad Spectrum of Neurological Conditions: A Cross-Sectional Nationally Representative Survey," *General Hospital Psychiatry* 37, no. 6 (2015): 507–12. https://doi.org/10.1016/j.genhosppsych.2015.06.007.

15. S. Goebel et al., "Distress in Patients with Newly Diagnosed Brain Tumours," *Psycho-Oncology* 20, no. 6 (2011): 623–30. https://doi.org/10.1002/pon.1958.

16. Brian Appleby, Kristin K. Appleby, and Peter V. Rabins, "Predictors of Depression and Anxiety in Patients with Intracranial Neoplasms," *Journal of Neuropsychiatry and Clinical Neurosciences* 20, no. 4 (2008): 447–49. https://doi.org/10.1176/jnp.2008.20.4.447.

17. Bendikt Habermeyer et al., "A Clinical Lesson: Glioblastoma Multiforme Masquerading as Depression in Chronic Alcoholic," *Alcohol and Alcoholism* 43, no. 1 (2008): 31–33. https://doi.org/10.1093/alcalc/agm150; Despina Moise and Subramoniam Madhusoodanan, "Psychiatric Symptoms Associated with Brain Tumors: A Clinical Enigma," *CNS Spectrums* 11, no. 1 (2006): 28–31. https://doi.org/10.1017/s1092852900024135.

18. Monika Janda et al., "Unmet Supportive Care Needs and Interests in Services among Patients with a Brain Tumour and Their Carers," *Patient Education and Counseling* 71, no. 2 (2008): 251–58. https://doi.org/10.1016/j.pec.2008.01.020.

19. C.P. Kaplan, and M. E. Miner, "Relationships: Importance for Patients with Cerebral Tumours," *Brain Injury* 14, no. 3 (2000): 251–59. https://doi.org/10.1080/026990500120727.

20. Monika Szpringer, Marzena Oledzka, and Benedikt L. Amann, "A Non-Randomized Controlled Trial of EMDR on Affective Symptoms in Patients With Glioblastoma Multiforme," *Frontiers in Psychology* 9 (May 2018): 785. https://doi.org/10.3389/fpsyg .2018.00785.

21. A.M. Bielecka, and E. Obuchowicz, "Antidepressant Drugs Can Modify Cytotoxic Action of Temozolomide," *European Journal of Cancer Care* 26, no. 5 (2017). https:// doi.org/10.1111/ecc.12551.

22. Rev. Diane Baldwin and Meredith Jones, "Developing an Acuity Tool to Optimize Nurse Navigation Caseloads," *Oncology Issues* 33, no. 2 (2018): 17–25. https://doi.org /10.1080/10463356.2018.1427983.

23. Larissa Nekhlyudov, Denalee M. O'Malley, and Shawna V Hudson, "Integrating Primary Care Providers in the Care of Cancer Survivors: Gaps in Evidence and Future Opportunities," *The Lancet Oncology* 18, no. 1 (2017): e30–38. https://doi.org /10.1016/S1470-2045(16)30570-8.

24. Office of Cancer Survivorship, "Statistics, Graphs and Definitions," *National Cancer Institute (NIH)*, accessed December 9, 2020, https://cancercontrol.cancer.gov/ocs /statistics#definitions.

25. Elyse R Park, Jeffrey Peppercorn, and Areej El-Jawahri, "Shades of Survivorship," *Journal of the National Comprehensive Cancer Network* 16, no. 10 (2018): 1163–65. https://doi.org/10.6004/jnccn.2018.7071.

26. Lynne S. Padgett, Kathleen Van Dyk, Natalie C. Kelly, Robin Newman, Sherry Hite, and Arash Asher, "Addressing Cancer-Related Cognitive Impairment in Cancer Survivorship," *Oncology Issues* 35, no. 1 (2020):52-57. https://doi.org/10.1080/10463356 .2020.1692601; Kimberly Stump-Sutliff, Louise Cunningham, and Todd Gersten, "Brain Tumors: Coping with Thinking and Memory Problems," *University of Rochester Medical Center,* n.d. https://www.urmc.rochester.edu/encyclopedia/content.aspx ?contenttypeid=34&contentid=18064-1.

27. Stacey L. Worrell et al., "Interdisciplinary Approaches to Survivorship with a Focus on the Low-Grade and Benign Brain Tumor Populations," *Current Oncology Reports* 23, no. 2 (2021): 19. https://doi.org/10.1007/s11912-020-01004-8.

28. Rudolph M. Navari, and Matti Aapro, "Antiemetic Prophylaxis for Chemotherapy-Induced Nausea and Vomiting," *The New England Journal of Medicine* 374, no. 14 (2016): 1356–67. https://doi.org/10.1056/NEJMra1515442.

29. Wolfgang Marx et al., "Chemotherapy-Induced Nausea and Vomiting: A Narrative Review to Inform Dietetics Practice," *Journal of the Academy of Nutrition and Dietetics* 116, no. 5 (2016): 819–27. https://doi.org/10.1016/j.jand.2015.10.020.

30. Ibid.

31. Nuriye Efe Ertürk, and Sultan Tasci, "The Effects of Peppermint Oil on Nausea, Vomiting and Retching in Cancer Patients Undergoing Chemotherapy: An Open Label Quasi-Randomized Controlled Pilot Study," *Complementary Therapies in*

Medicine 56 (January 2021): 102587. https://doi.org/10.1016/j.ctim.2020.102587; Jane T. Hickok et al., "A Phase II/III Randomized, Placebo-Controlled, Double-Blind Clinical Trial of Ginger (Zingiber Officinale) for Nausea Caused by Chemotherapy for Cancer: A Currently Accruing URCC CCOP Cancer Control Study," *Supportive Cancer Therapy* 4, no. 4 (2007): 247–50. https://doi.org/10.3816/SCT.2007.n.022.

32. J. M. Ezzo et al., "Acupuncture-Point Stimulation for Chemotherapy-Induced Nausea or Vomiting," *Cochrane Database System Review* no. 2 (April 2006): CD002285. https://doi.org/10.1002/14651858.CD002285.pub2.

33. Shelly Latte-Naor and Jun J. Mao, "Putting Integrative Oncology Into Practice: Concepts and Approaches," *Journal of Oncology Practice* 15, no. 7 (2019): 7–14. https://doi.org/10.1200/JOP.18.00554; Dina M. Randazzo et al., "Complementary and Integrative Health Interventions and Their Association with Health-Related Quality of Life in the Primary Brain Tumor Population," *Complementary Therapies in Clinical Practice* 36 (August 2009): 43–48. https://doi.org/10.1016/j.ctcp.2019.05.002; Farah Z. Zia et al., "The National Cancer Institute's Conference on Acupuncture for Symptom Management in Oncology: State of the Science, Evidence, and Research Gaps," *JNCI Monographs* 2017, no. 52 (2017): lgx005. https://doi.org/10.1093/jncimonographs/lgx005; Wendy Demark-Wahnefried et al., "Practical Clinical Interventions for Diet, Physical Activity, and Weight Control in Cancer Survivors," *CA: A Cancer Journal for Clinicians* 65, no. 3 (2015): 167–89. https://doi.org/10.3322/caac.21265; Arash Asher, Jack B. Fu, Charlotte Bailey, and Jennifer K. Hughes, "Fatigue among Patients with Brain Tumors," *CNS Oncology* 5, no. 2 (2016): 91–100. https://doi.org/10.2217/cns-2015-0008; Noël Arring, Debra L. Barton, Trevor Brooks, and Suzanna M. Zick, "Integrative Therapies for Cancer-Related Fatigue," *Cancer Journal* 25, no. 5 (2019): 349–56. https://doi.org/10.1097/PPO.0000000000000396

34. Diane E Meier et al., "A National Strategy For Palliative Care," *Health Affairs* 36, no. 7 (July 1, 2017): 1265–73, https://doi.org/10.1377/hlthaff.2017.0164.

35. "National Quality Forum," *National Quality Forum*, accessed May 10, 2021, https://www.qualityforum.org/Home.aspx.

36. Meier et al., "A National Strategy For Palliative Care."

37. Dio Kavalieratos et al., "Association Between Palliative Care and Patient and Caregiver Outcomes: A Systematic Review and Meta-Analysis," *Journal of American Medical Association* 316, no. 20 (November 22, 2016): 2104–14, https://doi.org/10.1001/jama.2016.16840.

38. Jennifer S. Temel et al., "Early Palliative Care for Patients with Metastatic Non-Small-Cell Lung Cancer," *The New England Journal of Medicine* 363 (2010): 733–42, https://doi.org/10.1056/NEJMoa1000678; Jessica J. Fulton et al., "Integrated Outpatient Palliative Care for Patients with Advanced Cancer: A Systematic Review and Meta-Analysis," *Palliative Care* 33, no. 2 (February 2019): 123–34, https://doi.org/10.1177/0269216318812633.

39. Havi Rosen et al., "The Benefit of Palliative Care on Brain Cancer Patients' Quality of Life" (2018): 532–35; Thomas Noh and Tobias Walbert, "Brain Metastasis: Clinical Manifestations, Symptom Management, and Palliative Care," *Handbook of Clinical Neurology* 149 (January 2018): 75-88; Eefje M Sizoo et al., "Symptoms and Problems in the End-of-Life Phase of High-Grade Glioma Patients," *Neuro-Oncology* 12, no. 11 (November 2010): 1162–66, https://doi.org/10.1093/neuonc/nop045.

40. Katerine LeMay and Keith G Wilson, "Treatment of Existential Distress in Life Threatening Illness: A Review of Manualized Interventions," *Clinical Psychology Review* 28, no. 3 (March 2008): 472–93; Kathleen E. Bickel et al., "An Integrative Framework of Appraisal and Adaptation in Serious Medical Illness" *Journal of Pain and Symptom Management* 60, no. 3 (September 2020): 657–77, https://doi.org/10.1016/j.jpainsymman.2020.05.018.

41. Meier et al., "A National Strategy For Palliative Care"; Dio Kavalieratos, "Directing the Narrative to Define and Present Standardization in Palliative Care," *Journal of Palliative Medicine* 22, no. 12 (December 2019): 1486–87, https://doi.org/10.1089/jpm.2019.0548.

42. M. Guzman et al., "A Pilot Clinical Study of Δ9-Tetrahydrocannabinol in Patients with Recurrent Glioblastoma Multiforme," *British Journal of Cancer* 95, no. 2 (2006): 197–203. https://doi.org/10.1038/sj.bjc.6603236.

43. Salim S Virani et al., "Heart Disease and Stroke Statistics-2021 Update: A Report From the American Heart Association," *Circulation* 143, no. 8 (February 23, 2021): e254–743, https://doi.org/10.1161/CIR.0000000000000950.

44. Magdalena Koszewicz et al., "Profile of Autonomic Dysfunctions in Patients with Primary Brain Tumor and Possible Autoimmunity," *Clinical Neurology and Neurosurgery* 151 (December 2016): 51–54, https://doi.org/10.1016/j.clineuro.2016.10.013.

45. National Institute of Health (NIH), "National Cancer Institute," *National Cancer Institute*, accessed September 27, 2021, https://www.cancer.gov/.

46. Patrick Y. Wen and Roger J. Packer, "The 2021 WHO Classification of Tumors of the Central Nervous System: Clinical Implications," *Neuro-Oncology* 23, no. 8 (2021): 1215–17, https://doi.org/10.1093/neuonc/noab120.

47. Claudia Scaringi, Linda Agolli, and Giuseppe Minniti, "Technical Advances in Radiation Therapy for Brain Tumors," *Anticancer Research* 38, no. 11 (November 2018): 6041-6045. https://doi.org/10.21873/anticanres.12954.

48. Kyle Wang and Joel E. Tepper, "Radiation Therapy-Associated Toxicity: Etiology, Management, and Prevention," *CA: A Cancer Journal for Clinicians* 71, no. 5 (September 2021): 437-454. https://doi.org/10.3322/caac.21689.

REFERENCES

Annegers, J. F., S. B. Shirts, W. A. Hauser, and L. T. Kurland. "Risk of Recurrence after an Initial Unprovoked Seizure." *Epilepsia* 27, no. 1 (February 1986): 43–50. https://doi.org/10.1111/j.1528-1157.1986.tb03499.x.

Appleby, Brian S., Kristin K. Appleby, and Peter V. Rabins. "Predictors of Depression and Anxiety in Patients with Intracranial Neoplasms." *Journal of Neuropsychiatry and Clinical Neurosciences* 20, no. 4 (2008): 447–49. https://doi.org/10.1176/jnp.2008.20.4.447.

Arif, Hiba, Richard Buchsbaum, Joanna Pierro, Michael Whalen, Jessica Sims, Stanley R. Resor Jr, Carl W. Bazil, and Lawrence J. Hirsch. "Comparative Effectiveness of 10 Antiepileptic Drugs in Older Adults with Epilepsy." *Archives of Neurology* 67, no. 4 (April 2010): 408–15. https://doi.org/10.1001/archneurol.2010.49.

Arring, Noël, Debra L. Barton, Trevor Brooks, and Suzanna M. Zick. "Integrative Therapies for Cancer-Related Fatigue." *Cancer Journal* 25, no. 5 (2019): 349–56. https://doi.org/10.1097/PPO.0000000000000396.

Asher, Arash, Jack B. Fu, Charlotte Bailey, and Jennifer K. Hughes. "Fatigue among Patients with Brain Tumors." *CNS Oncology* 5, no. 2 (2016): 91–100. https://doi.org/10.2217/cns-2015-0008.

Berg, Anne T. "Risk of Recurrence after a First Unprovoked Seizure." *Epilepsia* 49 (2008): 13–18. https://doi.org/10.1111/j.1528-1167.2008.01444.x.

Baldwin, Rev. Diane and Meredith Jones. "Developing an Acuity Tool to Optimize Nurse Navigation Caseloads." *Oncology Issues* 33, no. 2 (2018): 17–25. https://doir.org/10.1080/10463356.2018.1427983.

Bickel, Kathleen E., Cari Levy, Edward R. MacPhee, Keri Brenner, Jennifer S. Temel, Joanna J. Arch, Joseph A. Greer. "An Integrative Framework of Appraisal and Adaptation in Serious Medical Illness." *Journal of Pain and Symptom Management* 60, no. 3 (September 2020): 657–77, https://doi.org/10.1016/j.jpainsymman.2020.05.018.

Bielecka, A. M. and E. Obuchowicz. "Antidepressant Drugs Can Modify Cytotoxic Action of Temozolomide." *European Journal of Cancer Care* 26, no. 5 (2017). https://doi.org/10.1111/ecc.12551.

Bulloch, Andrew G. M., Kirsten M. Fiest, Jeanne V. A. Williams, Dina H. Lavorato, Sandra A. Berzins, Nathalie Jette, Tamara M. Pringsheim, and Scott B. Patten. "Depression—a Common Disorder across Broad Spectrum of Neurological Conditions: A Cross-Sectional Nationally Representative Survey." *General Hospital Psychiatry* 37, no. 6 (2015): 507–12. https://doi.org/10.1016/j.genhosppsych.2015.06.007.

Demark-Wahnefried, Wendy, Laura Q. Rogers, Catherine M. Alfano, Cynthia A. Thomson, Kerry S. Courneya, Jeffrey A. Meyerhardt, Nicole L. Stout, Elizabeth Kvale, Heidi Ganzer, and Jennifer A. Ligibel. "Practical Clinical Interventions for Diet, Physical Activity, and Weight Control in Cancer Survivors." *CA: A Cancer Journal for Clinicians* 65, no. 3 (2015): 167–89. https://doi.org/10.3322/caac.21265.

Ertürk, Nuriye Efe and Sultan Tasci. "The Effects of Peppermint Oil on Nausea, Vomiting and Retching in Cancer Patients Undergoing Chemotherapy: An Open Label Quasi-Randomized Controlled Pilot Study." *Complementary Therapies in Medicine* 56 (January 2021): 102587. https://doi.org/10.1016/j.ctim.2020.102587.

Ezzo, J. M., M. A. Richardson, A. Vickers, C. Allen, S. L. Dibble, B. F. Issell, L. Lao, M. Pearl, G. Ramirez, Ja Roscoe, J. Shen, J. C. Shivnan, K. Streitberger, I. Treish, G. Zhang. "Acupuncture-Point Stimulation for Chemotherapy-Induced Nausea or Vomiting." *Cochrane Database System Review* no. 2 (April 2006): CD002285. https://doi.org/10.1002/14651858.CD002285.pub2.

Fisher, Robert S., Carlos Acevedo, Alexis Arzimanoglou, Alicia Bogacz, J. Helen Cross, Christian E. Elger, Jerome Engel Jr., Lars Forsgren, Jacqueline A. French, Mike Glynn, Dale C. Hesdorffer, B.I. Lee, Gary W. Mathern, Solomon L. Moshé, Emilio Perucca, Ingrid E. Scheffer, Torbjörn Tomson, Masako Watanabe, and Samuel Wieber. "ILAE Official Report: A Practical Clinical Definition of Epilepsy." *Epilepsia* 55, no. 4 (April 2014): 475–82. https://doi.org/10.1111/epi.12550.

Fulton, Jessica J., Thomas W. LeBlanc, Toni M Cutson, Kathryn N. Porter Starr, Arif Kamal, Katherine Ramos, Caroline E. Freiermuth, Jennifer R. McDuffie, Andrzej Kosinski, Soheir Adam, Avishek Nagi, John W. Williams. "Integrated Outpatient Palliative Care for Patients with Advanced Cancer: A Systematic Review and Meta-Analysis." *Palliative Care* 33, no. 2 (February 2019): 123–34, https://doi.org/10.1177/0269216318812633.

Glantz, M. J., B. F. Cole, P. A. Forsyth, L. D. Recht, P. Y. Wen, M. C. Chamberlain, S. A. Grossman, and J. G. Cairncross. "Practice Parameter: Anticonvulsant Prophylaxis in Patients with Newly Diagnosed Brain Tumors. Report of the Quality Standards Subcommittee of the American Academy of Neurology." *Neurology* 54, no. 10 (May 23, 2000): 1886–93. https://doi.org/10.1212/wnl.54.10.1886.

Goebel, S., A.M. Stark, L. Kaup, M. von Harscher, and H.M. Mehdorn. 2011. "Distress in Patients with Newly Diagnosed Brain Tumours." *Psycho-Oncology* 20, no. 6 (2011): 623–30. https://doi.org/10.1002/pon.1958.

Guzman, M., M.J. Duarte, C. Blazque, J. Ravina, M.C. Rosa, I. Galve-Roperh, C. Sanchez, G. Velasco, and L. Gonzalez-Feria. "A Pilot Clinical Study of Δ9-Tetrahydrocannabinol in Patients with Recurrent Glioblastoma Multiforme." *British Journal of Cancer* 95, no. 2 (2006): 197–203. https://doi.org/10.1038/sj.bjc.6603236.

Habermeyer, Benedikt, Marcus Weiland, Ralf Mager, Gerhard A. Weisback, and Friedrich M. Wurst. "A Clinical Lesson: Glioblastoma Multiforme Masquerading as Depression in Chronic Alcoholic." *Alcohol and Alcoholism* 43, no. 1 (2008): 31–33. https://doi.org/10.1093/alcalc/agm150.

Hickok, Jane T., Joseph A. Roscoe, Gary R. Marrow, and Julie L. Ryan. "A Phase II/III Randomized, Placebo-Controlled, Double-Blind Clinical Trial of Ginger (Zingiber

Officinale) for Nausea Caused by Chemotherapy for Cancer: A Currently Accruing URCC CCOP Cancer Control Study." *Supportive Cancer Therapy* 4, no. 4 (2007): 247–50. https://doi.org/10.1093/alcalc/agm150.

Jallon, P., P. Loiseau, and J. Loiseau. "Newly Diagnosed Unprovoked Epileptic Seizures: Presentation at Diagnosis in CAROLE Study. Coordination Active Du Réseau Observatoire Longitudinal de l'Epilepsie." *Epilepsia* 42, no. 4 (April 2001): 464–75. https://doi.org/10.1046/j.1528-1157.2001.31400.x.

Janda, Monika, Suzanne Steginga, Jeff Dunn, Danette Langbecker, David Walker, and Elizabeth Eakin. "Unmet Supportive Care Needs and Interests in Services among Patients with a Brain Tumour and Their Carers." *Patient Education and Counseling* 71, no. 2 (2008): 251–58. https://doi.org/10.1016/j.pec.2008.01.020.

Kaplan, C. P. and M. E. Miner. "Relationships: Importance for Patients with Cerebral Tumours." *Brain Injury* 14, no. 3 (2000): 251–59. https://doi.org/10.1080/026990500120727.

Kavalieratos, Dio. "Directing the Narrative to Define and Present Standardization in Palliative Care." *Journal of Palliative Medicine* 22, no. 12 (December 2019): 1486–87, https://doi.org/10.1089/jpm.2019.0548.

Kavalieratos, Dio, Jennifer Corbelli, Di Zhang, J. Nicholas Dionne-Odom, Natalie C. Ernecoff, Janel Hanmer, Zachariah P. Hoydich, Dara Z. Ikejiani, Michele Klein-Fedyshin, Camilla Zimmermann, Sally C. Morton, Robert M. Arnold, Lucas Heller, and Yael Schenker. "Association Between Palliative Care and Patient and Caregiver Outcomes: A Systematic Review and Meta-Analysis." *Journal of American Medical Association* 316, no. 20 (November 22, 2016): 2104–14, https://doi.org/10.1001/jama.2016.16840.

Koszewicz, Magdalena, Slawomir Michalak, Malgorzata Bilinskaa, Slawomir Budrewicza, Mikolaj Zaborowskid, Krzysztof Slotwinskia, Ryszard Podemskia, and Maria Ejmaa. "Profile of Autonomic Dysfunctions in Patients with Primary Brain Tumor and Possible Autoimmunity." *Clinical Neurology and Neurosurgery* 151 (December 2016): 51–54, https://doi.org/10.1016/j.clineuro.2016.10.013.

Krumholz, Allan, Samuel Wiebe, Gary S. Gronseth, David S. Gloss, Ana M. Sanchez, Arif A. Kabir, Aisha T. Liferidge, Justin P. Martello, Andres M. Kanner, Shlomo Shinnar, Jennifer L. Hopp, and Jacqueline A. French. "Evidence-Based Guideline: Management of an Unprovoked First Seizure in Adults: Report of the Guideline Development Subcommittee of the American Academy of Neurology and the American Epilepsy Society." *Neurology* 84, no. 16 (April 21, 2015): 1705–13. https://doi.org/10.1212/WNL.0000000000001487.

Latte-Naor, Shelly and Jun J. Mao. "Putting Integrative Oncology Into Practice: Concepts and Approaches." *Journal of Oncology Practice* 15, no. 7 (2019): 7–14. https://doi.org/10.1200/JOP.18.00554.

LeMay, Katerine and Keith G Wilson. "Treatment of Existential Distress in Life

Threatening Illness: A Review of Manualized Interventions." *Clinical Psychology Review* 28, no. 3 (March 2008): 472–93.

Loughan, Ashlee R., Autumn Lanoye, Farah J. Aslanzadeh, Audrey Ann Lois Villanueva, Rachel Boutte, Mariya Husain, and Sarah Braun. "Fear of Cancer Recurrence and Death Anxiety: Unaddressed Concerns for Adult Neuro-Oncology Patients." *Journal of Clinical Psychology in Medical Settings* 28, no. 1 (2021): 16–30. https://doi.org/10.1007/s10880-019-09690-8.

Marx, Wolfgang, Nicole Kiss, Alexandra L McCarthy, Dan McKavanagh, and Liz Isenring. "Chemotherapy-Induced Nausea and Vomiting: A Narrative Review to Inform Dietetics Practice." *Journal of the Academy of Nutrition and Dietetics* 116, no. 5 (2016): 819–27. https://doi.org/10.1016/j.jand.2015.10.020.

Maschio, Marta, Francesca Sperati, Loredana Dinapoli, Antonello Vidiri, Alessandra Fabi, Andrea Pace, Alfredo Pompili, Carmine Maria Carapella, and Tonino Cantelmi. "Weight of Epilepsy in Brain Tumor Patients." *Journal of Neuro-Oncology* 118, no. 2 (May 2014): 385-393. https://doi.org/10.1007/s11060-014-1449-7.

Maschio, M., L. Dinapoli, S. Gomellini, V. Ferraresi, F. Sperati, A. Vidiri, P. Muti, and B. Jandolo. "Antiepileptics in Brain Metastases: Safety, Efficacy and Impact on Life Expectancy." *Journal of Neuro-Oncology* 98 (2009): 109–16. https://doi.org/10.1007/s11060-009-0069-0.

Maschio, Marta, Umberto Aguglia, Giuliano Avanzini, Paola Banfi, Carla Buttinelli, Giuseppe Capovilla, Marina Maria Luisa Casazza, Gabriella Colicchio, Antonietta Coppola, Cinzia Costa, Filippo Dainese, Ornella Daniele, Roberto De Simone, Marica Eoli, Sara Gasparini, Anna Teresa Giallonardo, Angela La Neve, Andrea Maialetti, Oriano Mecarelli, Marta Melis, Roberto Michelucci, Francesco Paladin, Giada Pauletto, Marta Piccioli, Stefano Quadri, Federica Ranzato, Rosario Rossi, Andrea Salmaggi, Riccardo Terenzi, Paolo Tisei, Flavio Villani, Paolo Vitali, Lucina Carla Vivalda, Gaetano Zaccara, Alessia Zarabla and Ettore Beghi. "Management of Epilepsy in Brain Tumors." *Neurological Sciences* 40, no. 10 (October 2019): 2217–34. https://doi.org/10.1007/s10072-019-04025-9.

Meier, Diane E., Anthony L. Back, Amy Berman, Susan D. Block, Janet M. Corrigan, and R. Sean Morrison. "A National Strategy for Palliative Care." *Health Affairs* 36, no. 7 (July 1, 2017): 1265–73, https://doi.org/10.1377/hlthaff.2017.0164.

Moise, Despina and Subramoniam Madhusoodanan. "Psychiatric Symptoms Associated with Brain Tumors: A Clinical Enigma." *CNS Spectrums* 11, no. 1 (2006): 28–31. https://doi.org/10.1017/s1092852900024135.

National Institute of Health (NIH). "National Cancer Institute." *National Cancer Institute*, accessed September 27, 2021. https://www.cancer.gov/.

"National Quality Forum." *National Quality Forum*, accessed May 10, 2021, https://www.qualityforum.org/Home.aspx.

Navari, Rudolph M. and Matti Aapro. "Antiemetic Prophylaxis for Chemotherapy-Induced Nausea and Vomiting." *The New England Journal of Medicine* 374, no. 14 (2016): 1356–67. https://doi.org/10.1056/NEJMra1515442.

Nekhlyudov, Larissa, Denalee M O'Malley, and Shawna V Hudson. "Integrating Primary Care Providers in the Care of Cancer Survivors: Gaps in Evidence and Future Opportunities." *The Lancet Oncology* 18, no. 1 (2017): e30–38. https://doi.org/10.1016/S1470-2045(16)30570-8.

Noh, Thomas and Tobias Walbert. "Brain Metastasis: Clinical Manifestations, Symptom Management, and Palliative Care." *Handbook of Clinical Neurology* 149 (January 2018): 75-88.

Office of Cancer Survivorship. "Statistics, Graphs and Definitions." *National Cancer Institute (NIH)*, accessed December 9, 2020. https://cancercontrol.cancer.gov/ocs/statistics#definitions.

Padgett, Lynne S., Kathleen Van Dyk, Natalie C. Kelly, Robin Newman, Sherry Hite, and Arash Asher. "Addressing Cancer-Related Cognitive Impairment in Cancer Survivorship." *Oncology Issues* 35, no. 1 (2020): 52-57. https://doi.org/10.1080/10463356.2020.1692601.

Park, Elyse R., Jeffrey Peppercorn, and Areej El-Jawahri. "Shades of Survivorship." *Journal of the National Comprehensive Cancer Network* 16, no. 10 (2018): 1163–65. https://doi.org/10.6004/jnccn.2018.7071.

Perucca. Emilio. "Clinically Relevant Drug Interactions with Antiepileptic Drugs." *British Journal of Clinical Pharmacology* 61, no. 3 (March 2006): 246–55. https://doi.org/10.1111/j.1365-2125.2005.02529.x.

Randazzo, Dina M., Frances McSherry, James E. Herndon, Mary L. Affronti, Eric S. Lipp, Charlene Flahiff, Elizabeth Miller, Sarah Woodring, Susan Boulton, Annick Desjardins, David M. Ashley, Henry S. Friedman, and Katherine B. Peters. "Complementary and Integrative Health Interventions and Their Association with Health-Related Quality of Life in the Primary Brain Tumor Population." *Complementary Therapies in Clinical Practice* 36 (August 2009): 43–48. https://doi.org/10.1016/j.ctcp.2019.05.002.

Rosen, Havi, Rikesh Patel, Soma Sengupta, and Ali Zarrabi. "The Benefit of Palliative Care on Brain Cancer Patients' Quality of Life," (2018): 532–35.

Scaringi, Claudia, Linda Agolli, and Giuseppe Minniti. "Technical Advances in Radiation Therapy for Brain Tumors." *Anticancer Research* 38, no. 11 (November 2018): 6041-6045. https://doi.org/10.21873/anticanres.12954.

Sizoo, Eefje M., Lies Braam, Tjeerd J. Postma, H. Roeline W. Pasman, Jan J. Heimans, Martin Klein, Jaap C. Reijneveld, and Martin J. B. Taphoorn "Symptoms and Problems in the End-of-Life Phase of High-Grade Glioma Patients." *Neuro-Oncology* 12, no. 11 (November 2010): 1162–66, https://doi.org/10.1093/neuonc/nop045.

Starkweather, Angela R., Paula Sherwood, Debra E. Lyon, Nancy L. McCain, Dana H. Bovbjerg, and William C Broaddus. "A Biobehavioral Perspective on Depressive Symptoms in Patients with Cerebral Astrocytomas." *Journal of Neuroscience Nursing* 43, no. 1 (2011): 17–28. https://doi.org/10.1097/jnn.0b013e3182029859.

Stump-Sutliff, Kimberly, Louise Cunningham, and Todd Gersten. "Brain Tumors: Coping with Thinking and Memory Problems." *University of Rochester Medical Center* (n.d.). https://www.urmc.rochester.edu/encyclopedia/content.aspx?contenttypeid =34&contentid=18064-1.

Szpringer, Monika, Marzena Oledzka, and Benedikt L. Amann. "A Non-Randomized Controlled Trial of EMDR on Affective Symptoms in Patients With Glioblastoma Multiforme." *Frontiers in Psychology* 9 (May 2018): 785. https://doi.org/10.3389/fpsyg .2018.00785.

Temel, Jennifer S., Joseph A. Greer, Alona Muzikansky, Emily R. Gallagher, Sonal Admane, Vicki A. Jackson, Constance M. Dahlin, Craig D. Blinderman, Juliet Jacobsen, William F. Pirl, J. Andrew Billings, and Thomas J. Lynch. "Early Palliative Care for Patients with Metastatic Non-Small-Cell Lung Cancer." *The New England Journal of Medicine* 363 (2010): 733–42, https://doi.org/10.1056/NEJMoa1000678.

Tremont-Lukats, I. W., B. O. Ratilal, T. Armstrong, and M. R. Gilbert. "Antiepileptic Drugs for Preventing Seizures in People with Brain Tumors." *Cochrane Database System Review* no. 2 (April 16, 2008): CD004424. https://doi.org/10.1002/14651858 .CD004424.pub2.

University of Rochester Medical Center. "Brain Tumors: Coping with Thinking and Memory Problems." In *Adult and Children's Health Encyclopedia*. https://www .urmc.rochester.edu/encyclopedia/content.aspx?contenttypeid=34&contentid =18064-1.

Vecht, Charles J. and Erik B. Wilms. "Seizures in Low- and High-Grade Gliomas: Current Management and Future Outlook." *Expert Review of Anticancer Therapy* 10, no. 5 (May 2010): 663–69. https://doi.org/10.1586/era.10.48.

Virani, Salim S., Alvaro Alonso, Hugo J. Aparicio, Emelia J. Benjamin, Marcio S. Bittencourt, Clifton W. Callaway, April P. Carson, Alanna M. Chamberlain, Susan Cheng, Francesca N. Delling, Mitchell S.V. Elkind, Kelly R. Evenson, Jane F. Ferguson, Deepak K. Gupta, Sadiya S. Khan, Brett M. Kissela, Kristen L. Knutson, Chong D. Lee, Tené T. Lewis, Junxiu Liu, Matthew Shane Loop, Pamela L. Lutsey, Jun Ma, Jason Mackey, Seth S. Martin, David B. Matchar, Michael E. Mussolino, Sankar D. Navaneethan, Amanda Marma Perak, Gregory A. Roth, Zainab Samad, Gary M. Satou, Emily B. Schroeder, Svati H. Shah, Christina M. Shay, Andrew Stokes, Lisa B. VanWagner, Nae-Yuh Wang, and Connie W Tsao, "Heart Disease and Stroke Statistics-2021 Update: A Report From the American Heart Association." *Circulation* 143, no. 8 (February 23, 2021): e254–743, https://doi.org/10.1161/ CIR.0000000000000950.

Wang, Kyle and Joel E. Tepper. "Radiation Therapy-Associated Toxicity: Etiology, Management, and Prevention." *CA: A Cancer Journal for Clinicians* 71, no. 5 (September 2021): 437-454. https://doi.org/10.3322/caac.21689.

Worrell, Stacey L., Michelle L. Kirschner, Rhonna S. Shatz, Soma Sengupta, and Melissa G. Erickson. "Interdisciplinary Approaches to Survivorship with a Focus on the Low-Grade and Benign Brain Tumor Populations." *Current Oncology Reports* 23, no. 2 (2021): 19. https://doi.org/10.1007/s11912-020-01004-8.

Wellisch, David K., Thomas A. Kaleita, Donald Freeman, Timothy Coughesy, and Jeffrey Goldman. "Predicting Major Depression in Brain Tumor Patients." *Psycho-Oncology* 11, no. 3 (2002): 230–38. https://doi.org/10.1002/pon.562.

Wen, Patrick Y. and Roger J. Packer. "The 2021 WHO Classification of Tumors of the Central Nervous System: Clinical Implications." *Neuro-Oncology* 23, no. 8 (2021): 1215–17, https://doi.org/10.1093/neuonc/noab120.

Wyllie, Elaine. "Encephalopathic Generalized Epilepsy and Lennox-Gastaut Syndrome." In *Wyllie's Treatment of Epilepsy: Principles and Practice*, 6th edition., 272–83. Philadelphia, PA: Wolters Kluwer, 2015.

Zia, Farah Z., Oluwadamilola Olaku, Ting Bao, Ann Berger, Gary Deng, Arthur Yin Fan, Mary K. Garcia, Patricia M. Herman, Ted J. Kaptchuk, Elena J. Ladas, Helene M. Langevin, Lixing Lao, Weidong Lu, Vitaly Napadow, Richard C. Niemtzow, Andrew J. Vickers, Xin Shelley Wang, Claudia M. Witt, and Jun J. Mao. "The National Cancer Institute's Conference on Acupuncture for Symptom Management in Oncology: State of the Science, Evidence, and Research Gaps," *JNCI Monographs* 2017, no. 52 (2017): lgx005. https://doi.org/10.1093/jncimonographs/lgx005.

EPILOGUE

From the various journeys of each patient, family member, and physician who appear in this book, there is an important overall lesson —there is no "one size fits all" in the care of any brain tumor patient. This book is not intended to be an exhaustive discussion of the science of each type of brain tumor, but rather the book's goal is to humanize how a patient's journey involves their families and providers. A beloved quote from Martin Luther King Jr. embodies the hope of brain tumor patients and their support teams— "We must accept finite disappointment, but never lose infinite hope."

There are many different types of brain tumors and presentations. There are benign brain tumors, malignant brain tumors, and tumors that affect the spinal cord. It is important for family members and medical professionals to truly listen to the patient and not label them simply as a medical case. As shown in this book, every individual's journey is different. The many stories in this book—an actor who regained his will to work; a veteran whose legacy lives on through his art; a nurse with a passion for music; a mother who had her balance restored; a young mother and nurse who fiercely loved her children; a woman who's genetic disorder gave her the determination to face adversity; a transgender individual who was able to continue on their gender-confirming process; a "sock-lover" who battled with her hearing loss; and a woman who sought help for her vision and memory issues—show the diversity in patient journeys with brain tumors and the value of support from friends, family, and medical providers.

This is not a book about cures. The case studies and compendium in this book instead highlight resources and perspectives that optimize care. The stories and individuals in the book show that it truly takes a village to take care of brain tumor patients. The contributors to this project hope that in a small way, they can introduce a resource for patients, families, and providers not in the specialty that helps them navigate treatment options.

GLOSSARY

5-Aminolevulinic acid (5-ALA): a natural chemical within the body that is produced during blood cell creation; used by neurosurgeons during surgery as a real-time marker of tumor boundaries for more accurate resection; currently being studied for light activation to selectively kill cancer

Acupuncture: an alternative form of medicine in which mechanical stimulation, electrical stimulation, or heat are used to stimulate body areas

Adjuvant: after initial cancer treatment

Alkylating agent: compounds or drugs that damage the DNA of cancer cells so that they cannot grow or divide

Amygdala: a part of the brain found in the temporal lobe that controls emotion, particularly fear and aggression

Anaphylactic: related to an allergic reaction

Anosmia: a partial or complete loss of smell

Anterior: near the front in position (i.e., the kneecap is on the anterior side of the leg)

Anterolateral: a combination of two anatomical localization terms (see **Anterior** and **Lateral**)

Anti-angiogenic: interrupts tumors' blood supply by preventing the formation of blood vessels

Anti-seizure medication (ASM): medication prescribed to treat focal epilepsy only

Antineoplastic: a classification of drugs that are used to treat cancer

Antipsychotic: a class of medication used to treat psychosis

Anxiety: a psychological condition used to describe intense worrying or fear

Aphasia: inability to create or understand speech

Art therapy: the utilization of art as a therapeutic modality

Astrocytoma: a type of brain or spinal cord tumor that arises from astrocytes

Asymptomatic: not experiencing symptoms

Ataxic: uncoordinated movement

Auditory brainstem implant (ABI): a surgically implanted device that restores hearing to people with hearing loss; a device that uses an electrode to create signals for the auditory nerve

Basal cell carcinoma (BCC): a common form of skin cancer with low metastatic potential; UV radiation is the most significant risk factor for BCC

Base pair: a unit of DNA

Belinostat (BELIODAQ®): a histone deacetylase drug

Benign: a descriptor for an abnormal growth that does not spread to other parts of the body and is noncancerous

Bevacizumab (AVASTIN®): an anti-angiogenic chemotherapy drug

Bifrontal craniotomy: a surgical procedure where the forehead and top of the head portions of the skull are opened to reach the brain

Biopsy: an examination of a sample of tissue taken from the body to be examined by a pathologist; can give insight into key molecular markers for different tumor subtypes

Birthmark: a skin abnormality that is present at birth

Bitemporal hemianopsia: loss of the outer half of each visual field in both eyes

Blood clot: coagulation of blood that may restrict blood flow within the vascular system

Brainstem: a structure that connects the bottom portion of the brain to the top of the spinal cord; contains brain centers that are critical to the maintenance of life (breathing, thirst, hunger, etc.)

Brivaracetam (BRIVIACT®, BRIVAZEN®): a medication that is used to treat partial seizures

Broca's area: area of the brain located in the frontal lobe that is responsible for the production of speech

Cachexia: a wasting syndrome where a patient experiences weight and muscle loss

Carbamazepine (TEGRETOL®): an anti-seizure medication that can have a strong effect on drug metabolism

Cardiology: medical specialization associated with the heart and vascular system

Cataract: Clouding of the naturally clear lens of the eye

Central nervous system: the brain, spinal cord, and associated connective tissue

Cerebellar hemisphere: the left or right divisions on either side of the vermis

Cerebellum: a part of the brain that coordinates muscular activity and balance

Cerebral blood volume (CBV): The amount of intravascular blood within a specific area of brain tissue; can be helpful in determining extent of damage to a brain area

Cerebral cortex: the outer layer of the brain

Cerebrum: largest part of the brain, located superiorly and anteriorly in relation to the brainstem

Cervical spine: the area of the spine in the region of the back of the neck

Charley horse: a term used to describe cramping

Chemoradiation: a term used to describe chemotherapy and radiation in combination to treat cancer

Chemotherapy: treatment of a disease, such as cancer, using chemical substances

Chordoid glioma: a rare intraventricular tumor which may arise in the third ventricle

Choroidal fissure: a c-shaped cleft in the brain that is directly above the hypothalamus

Chronic: lasting for a long time

Clinical trial: research studies used to investigate medical intervention; typically involves multiple stages during which the proposed therapeutic undergoes extensive safety, dosing, and efficacy testing

Cochlear implant: a surgically implanted electronic device that stimulates the cochlear nerve to aid hearing

Cognition: mental processes involved in thinking, learning, knowledge, and being self-aware

Comorbid: conditions that occur simultaneously or at the same time

Computed tomography (CT): series of x-rays taken together to yield a detailed 3D image

Concussion: a brain injury caused by trauma to the head

Consortium to Establish a Registry for Alzheimer's Disease (CERAD): a verbal cognitive assessment given by a medical professional to test evaluate cognitive abilities

Coronal: A vertical plane which divides the body into anterior and posterior.

Corticospinal tract (CST): tract that consists of axons which carry motor control information from the brain to the spinal cord

Craniopharyngioma: rare, benign tumor located within the skull that results from cancerous transformation of Rathke's pouch

Craniotomy: surgical opening of the skull to reach the brain

Cystic: resembling a cyst; abnormal pocket-like area of tissue

Cytopenia: low blood counts

Deaf: complete loss of hearing

Debulk: remove as much of the bulk of tumor as possible

Dentist: a specialist in oral care and teeth

Depression: a psychological condition defined as a persistent feeling of sadness and loss of interest

Dermatology: a field of medicine that specializes in skin

Desensitization: gradually increasing the dose of chemotherapy drug to avoid negative reactions

Dexamethasone (DECADRON®): a steroid used to decrease inflammation

Diabetes insipidus: disease in which the body cannot regulate how it handles fluids due to issues with the production or reception of the hormone, ADH, causing intense thirst and heavy urination; common complication of craniopharyngioma surgery when the pituitary stalk must be cut to remove all the tumor

Diabetes mellitus: a disease in which the body has lost its ability to produce or respond to insulin, causing abnormal metabolism and elevated glucose levels in the blood and urine

Dura mater: tough outermost layer of the meninges covering the brain and spinal cord

Dysmetria: problems with controlling speed and range of motion needed to perform coordinated movements when judging distance to a target

Dyspnea: difficulty breathing

Edema: swelling due to fluid accumulation

Electrocardiogram (EKG): a medical test that measures the electrical activity in the heart to identify heart conditions

Electroencephalogram (EEG): a medical test that measures the electrical activity in the brain; commonly used to diagnose epileptic conditions

Endocrine: a system of glands that produce hormones regulating metabolism, growth and development, tissue function, sexual function, reproduction, sleep, mood, and other areas of human behavior

Enhancing lesion: an area that appears bright on MRI due to increased uptake of the contrast agent gadolinium; enhancement typically denotes increased vascularity

Enzyme: a protein responsible for speeding up a biochemical reaction

Ependymal: pertaining to the inner lining of the ventricles

Epidermal growth factor receptor (EGFR): receptor involved in cell growth

Epilepsy: a brain condition that results in seizures

Epileptologist: a physician who specializes in epilepsy

Executive function: mental skills such as memory, attention, and planning that are used to manage daily life

Existential distress: describes the psychological distress that is felt when faced with the possibility of death

Eye movement desensitization and reprocessing (EMDR): a psychotherapy treatment used to alleviate stress

Family medicine: a branch of medicine within primary care that focuses on treating people of all ages and genders

Fatigue: tiredness

Fibroblast growth factor receptor (FGFR): cellular receptors that are important for cell growth and distinction

Focal seizure: a seizure that begins in one area of the brain

Foot drop: the inability to pick up the front of the foot which can cause one's foot to drag on the ground during walking

Frontal horn: A subdivision of the lateral ventricles which extends anteriorly from the foramen of Monro

Frontal lobe: major lobe in the front part of the cerebral cortex that regulates higher order function

Fusiform face area: a part of the visual system in the brain that is responsible for recognizing faces

Gait: limb movements made during walking

Gastroesophageal reflux disease (GERD): acid reflux disease that occurs when stomach acid flows up into the esophagus and irritates the outer cell lining.

Gastrointestinal: a system of the body which consists of the stomach and intestines

Gender: the behavioral characteristics of women, men, girls, and boys, that are socially constructed

Gene regulation: mechanisms that control gene expression

Gene: a hereditary unit which is passed from generation to generation and the expression of which can manifest as a physical characteristic

Generalized tonic-clonic seizure: a type of seizure that occurs due to disturbance in both hemispheres of the brain; loss of consciousness and violent muscle contractions are common presentations

Germ cell: a cell that contributes to gonad formation in sexually reproducing organisms

Glaucoma: increased pressure within the eyeball resulting in the loss of sight

Glioblastoma multiforme: a malignant tumor that arises from glial cells (see **accessory/ glial cell**) in the brain; a very common adult primary brain tumor

Gout: a disease characterized by arthritis, especially in the feet; the abnormal metabolism of uric acid creates crystals that deposit in joints causing episodes of acute pain

Gross total resection: surgical removal of all the tumor as defined on MRI

Hemisphere (left or right): halves of the brain

Hippocampus: structure in temporal lobe that plays a key role in learning and memory

Histone deacetylase (HDAC) inhibitor: a class of drug used to alter gene expression of cancer cells, instigating their death

Histone protein: proteins that help support the structure of chromosomes

Hormones: class of signaling molecules produced by endocrine glands that are transported in blood vessels to regulate human bodily functions and behavior

Hospice: a branch of healthcare focused on providing palliative care to patients toward the end of life

Hydrocephalus: abnormal buildup of fluid in the ventricles

Hyperglycemia: high blood sugar levels

Hypertension: elevated blood pressure

Hyponatremia: low blood sodium

Hypothalamus: a brain region that secretes certain hormones, body temperature, hunger, thirst, sleep, and some emotional activity

Hysterectomy: surgical removal of the uterus

Immunotherapy: a form of cancer treatment that helps the immune system fight off cancer

Inflammation: pain or swelling due to white blood cells responding to a harmful infection

Insomnia: a sleep disorder in which it is difficult to fall and stay asleep

Integrative medicine: a specialty of medicine which focuses on the entire person to achieve health and healing

Intensity modulated radiation therapy (IMRT): a type of therapy typically that delivers a precise low dose of radiation to a tumor Intracranial: inside of the skull

Intraocular: inside of the eye

Intravenous (IV): inside of the vein

Intraventricular: inside of the ventricle

Isocitrate dehydrogenase (IDH) mutant: a classification of tumor based off molecular characteristics; normal IDH is expressed within cells and plays a role in metabolism, however, when IDH is mutated, it leads to genetic changes which have the capability of promoting tumor growth; mutant suggests there is a mutation in the function of the IDH protein which is common in low-grade gliomas or secondary GBMs

Isocitrate dehydrogenase (IDH) wild-type: a classification of tumor based off molecular characteristics; wild-type suggests primary GBMs

Lacosamide (VIMPAT®): an anti-convulsant medication

Lamotrigine (LAMICTAL®): an anti-seizure medication

Lateral: toward the side (i.e., the arms are lateral to the chest)

Letrozole (FEMARA®): a hormone-based chemotherapy drug that reduces the amount of estrogen in the body to treat breast cancer

Levetiracetam (KEPPRA®): an anti-seizure medication

Limbic cortex: area of the brain where several important structures are located, which function to control emotion, behavior, and long-term memory

Lomustine (GLEOSTINE®): an anti-cancer alkylating chemotherapy drug (see **alkylating agent**)

Magnetic Resonance Imaging (MRI): a form of medical imaging that uses a strong magnetic field and radio waves to produce images of the internal organs; helpful for the determining the extent of resection in gross total resection (see **resection, gross total resection**)

Magnetic resonance spectroscopic imaging (MRSI): imaging that uses strong magnetic field and radio waves to measure biochemical changes within the brain

Maintenance therapy: cancer care that is given to prolong remission

Malignant: cancerous; cells that spread to other parts of the body

Mass effect: effects of a growing mass that pushes on or displaces surrounding tissue

Massage therapy: a therapeutic mechanism of rubbing muscles

Mediterranean diet: a diet inspired by foods and eating habits of those living near the Mediterranean Sea; diet traditionally includes lots of fruits, vegetables, beans and whole grains with a scarcity of red meat; has been associated with better outcomes with cancer-related symptoms.

Melanoma: a form of skin cancer with common metastases to the brain

Meninges: three membranes that line the skull and vertebral canal to enclose the brain and spinal cord; from closest to the brain to the skull: pia mater, arachnoid, dura mater

Meningioma(s): benign tumor(s) arising from the meningeal tissue of the brain

Meta-analysis: a research design that analyzes data produced from several published studies

Microenvironment: the environment that surrounds and supports cells

Mindfulness meditation: meditation focusing on the state of being conscious

Music therapy: the utilization of music as a therapeutic modality

Mutation: an alteration causing change

Myelin: a substance composed of lipids that surrounds the axons of nerves to insulate them; this insulation helps speed up the electrical conductance of axons similar in theory to insulating copper electrical wiring

National Institute of Health (NIH): a medical research center of the U.S. government

Nausea: stomach discomfort resulting in the feeling of needing to vomit; the feeling of nausea is a common side effect of chemotherapy thought to be an effect of overstimulation of the area postrema within the brain

Neocortex: the part of the brain responsible for higher thinking and function such as decision-making

Neoplasm: an abnormal growth of cells in the body

Neuro-oncologist: a physician who specialized in treating brain tumors with medical therapy; coordinates care among the various specialists involved in brain tumor treatment

Neuroanatomist: an expert who studies the anatomy of the brain

Neurocognition: a term used to describe cognition and how it is impacted by the brain

Neurocognitive: the brain's structures and processes as they relate to cognition

Neurofibroma: small benign nerve growths

Neurofibromatosis type 1 (NF1): a genetic condition that predisposes patients to developing tumors along nerves; clinical presentation includes light brown skin spots and benign skin tumors (see **Neurofibroma**)

Neurofibromatosis type 2 (NF2): a genetic disease that causes tumors to form from nerve cell sheaths throughout the body; clinically presents with an increased prevalence of bilateral vestibular schwannoma (see **vestibular schwannoma**)

Neurologist: a physician specializing in the anatomy, function, and disorders of the nerves and nervous system

Neurology: field of medicine involved in the treatment of diseases of the brain, spinal cord, and nervous system without surgery

Neurons: fundamental cells of the brain and nervous system

Neuropathy: damage to nerve endings that can manifest as pain, weakness, and/or numbness depending on the nerves involved

Neuropsychologist: a psychologist that focuses on behavior and its relation to the brain

Neurosurgeon: a surgeon who specializes in surgery of the nervous system, especially the brain and spinal cord

Neurotologist: a physician who specializes in neurological related inner ear issues

NIH Toolbox Cognition Battery: an application-based cognitive assessment administered to test cognitive abilities

Nurse navigator: a nursing professional that assists patients through the course of their diagnosis, treatment, and survivorship

O[6]-methylguanine-DNA methyltransferase (MGMT): a DNA repair enzyme; methylation of this enzyme in cancer cells inactivates it and reduces DNA repair abilities of cancer cells; this genetic modification confers a favorable outcome when using alkylating agents

Occipital lobe: most posterior lobe of the brain; responsible for vision processing

Occupational therapy (OT): a branch of healthcare that focuses on treating physical, sensory, and cognitive issues

Olanzapine (ZYPREXA®): an antipsychotic medication

Olfactory groove meningiomas (OGMs): benign tumors that form between the nose and the eyebrow area at the front part of the skull

Olfactory groove: the area of the skull between the nose and the eyebrow

Oligodendrocytes: a type of cell that provides support and myelination to nerves within the central nervous system (see **myelin**)

Oncology: a medical specialty that focuses on the treatment of cancer

Ophthalmologist: a physician who specializes in the anatomy, function, and disorders of the eye

Optic chiasm: crossing of optic nerves that carry visual signals from the outer half of both the left and right visual fields

Optic nerve: special nerve in the back of each eye that transfers visual information from the retina to the vision centers of the brain via electrical impulses

Optune® device: a form of cancer treatment that uses electrical fields to stop cancer cells from growing or dividing; it resembles a thin, white cap that is worn on the head

Ovarian cancer: cancer in the female reproductive organ ovary

Overactive bladder: condition where there are frequent or sudden urges to urinate

Oxcarbazepine (TRILEPTAL®): an anti-seizure medication; anti-convulsant medication

Parahippocampal gyrus: area that surrounds the hippocampus that plays an important role in spatial awareness

Parahippocampal place area: a part of the brain responsible for scene or place recognition

Paresthesia: burning or prickling sensation in an extremity

Parietal lobe: major lobe in the upper back part of the cerebral cortex that processes sensory information

Pathology: the typical features or behaviors of a disease; a field of medicine dedicated to the cause and nature of disease

PD-1/PD-L1 pathway: a cellular pathway that maintains immune tolerance within the cancer cell

Pediatrician: a physician who treats children

Peri-: around

Peripheral nervous system (PNS): the nervous system outside of the brain and spinal cord

Phenobarbital (SOLFOTON®): an anti-seizure medication that can have a strong effect on drug metabolism

Phenytoin (DILANTIN®): an anti-seizure medication that has a strong effect on drug metabolism

Photon: an electromagnetic radiation particle Pineal **region**: posterior to the third ventricle

Pituitary gland: pea-shaped gland on the base of the brain that controls multiple functions of the human body, including digestion, sexuality, and the body's response to stress

Pituitary stalk: connection between the pituitary gland and the brain

Pons: a major division of the brainstem which contains ascending and descending neuronal tracts implicated in a wide range of processes

Pontine angle cistern: a CSF-filled space that lies anteriorly to the cerebellum and lateral to the pons; clinically important as it is a common localization of multiple tumors

Posterior: further back in position (i.e., the back is posterior to the chest)

Postoperative: after surgery

Posttraumatic stress disorder (PTSD): a psychological disorder stemming from a traumatic event that is experienced in a person's life

Premorbid: occurring before diseases

Primary auditory cortex: a part of the brain, located in the temporal lobe, that is responsible for identifying pitch and sound

Primary brain tumor: tumors that originate within the brain

Primary care physician: a physician who practices preventative care; often this includes conducting routine physicals, annual appointments, or screenings

Primary intraventricular tumor: a tumor that stays within the third ventricle

Primary motor cortex: the most important area of the cerebral cortex for producing motor movements; located in the frontal lobe

Primidone (MYSOLINE®): an anti-seizure medication that can have a strong effect on drug metabolism

Probiotics: live microorganisms that promote digestive health

Prognosis: the likely outcome of a situation

Proinflammatory cytokines: regulatory molecules secreted by cells of the immune system that favor inflammation

Proximal: toward the center of the body (i.e., the shoulder is proximal to the hand)

Psychosocial: involving social and psychological aspects

Quetiapine (SEROQUEL®): an antipsychotic medication

Radiation mask: a plastic-like mold or cast that is uniquely made to fit a patient to keep their head and neck in place for accurate delivery of radiation therapy

Radiation oncologist: a physician who specializes in radiation as treatment for cancer

Radiation oncology: a medical specialty that focuses on radiation therapy

Radiation plan: a medical plan created by radiation oncologists and radiation oncology staff to determine where radiation will be given to a patient

Radiation planning scan: a CT scan that radiation oncologists use to identify where radiation should be given based on the tumor's location

Radiation therapy/radiotherapy: cancer treatment that uses beams of intense energy to kill cancer cells

Radiosurgery: focused beam of radiation therapy

Recurrent: returning; coming back

Resection: surgical removal

Respiratory system: a set of organs dedicated to the task of gas exchange with the environment

Retrospective chart review: a research design that uses patient information in medical records to investigate a scientific question

Sagittal: an anatomical plane longitudinally through the middle of the body which splits the body into a left and right half.

Schwann cells: cells that myelinate axons in the peripheral nervous system

Schwannoma: a nerve sheath tumor that originates from Schwann cells

Scoliosis: sideways curvature of the spine

Secondary intraventricular tumor: a tumor that grows adjacent to the third ventricle or the suprasellar region and spreads into the third ventricle as it grows

Seizure: uncontrolled electrical activity within the brain resulting in temporary uncontrollable muscle movements or consciousness

Serotonergic antidepressants: a form of medication that increases serotonin levels to combat depression

Sex: male or female assignment at birth

Shunt: a passageway made by surgery to redirect fluid to another area of the body; used to treat hydrocephalus

Sinus infection: an infection in the lining of the sinus cavity

Skull base: junction of where the brain meets the face

Social worker: a professional that assists patients in solving and coping with challenges from life, such as unemployment, access to care, and familial issues

Spatial memory: recalling information related to space and location; main processing center is the hippocampus

Speech therapy: an area of healthcare focused on treating speech related issues

Spinal column: the spine; bones, muscles and tissues that surround the spinal cord

Spinal cord: a long, tube-like structure that begins in the brain stem and ends near the bottom of the spine; transmits information from the brain to the rest of the body

Stereotactic radio surgery (SRS): an extremely precise form of radiation treatment

Superior: toward the head (i.e. the nose is superior to the mouth)

Suprasellar: situated or rising above the sella turcica which is a saddle-like bony prominence in the middle of the inferior skull that houses the pituitary gland; used to anatomically reference tumors of the pituitary gland

Survivorship: the period of time where a patient is surviving cancer

Suture: surgical threading used to sew incisions closed

T-cells: a component of the immune system that recognizes foreign substances

Tai chi: a form of martial arts

Temozolomide (TMZ, TEMODAR®): a DNA alkylator medication

Temporal lobe: the part of the brain that sits behind the ears; responsible for hearing, visual processes, identifying objects, and navigation

Testosterone: a male sex hormone

Therapeutic profile: the types of therapeutic options that can be used for healthcare treatment

Third ventricle: one of four connected ventricles in the brain's ventricular system; it is filled with cerebrospinal fluid

Topiramate (TOPOMAX®): a medication used to prevent seizures

Trans-choroidal fissure: an approach to the 3rd ventricle via opening the taenia fornicis of the choroid fissure and proceeding between the two internal cerebral veins

Transducer arrays: contain ceramic discs that create tumor treating fields for the Optune® device

Transgender: a characterization for when a person's gender identity does not match to the sex they were assigned at birth

Traumatic brain injury (TBI): a brain injury that is caused by a traumatic event that occurs to the head

Tumor treating fields (TTFs): electrical fields that can interfere with cancer cell division and replication (see **Optune® device**)

Urinary incontinence: loss of bladder control; can be a by-product of spinal cord impairment which allows clinicians to localize neurological issues

Urinary tract infection (UTI): an infection of the urinary system

Valproic acid (DEPAKENE®): an anti-convulsant medication prescribed to treat epilepsy or bipolar disorder

Vascular endothelial growth factor protein (VEGF): a protein that functions to signal the creation of new blood vessels; this is a common target for cancer therapy given that growing cancer cells require an extensive blood vessel network

Vermis: the central portion of the cerebellum that is responsible for coordinating movements closer to the trunk of the body

Vestibular schwannoma (VS): also termed acoustic neuroma; benign tumor of the Schwann cells surrounding CN VIII

Vestibulocochlear nerve (CN VIII): cranial nerve VIII; carries information of hearing and balance from the inner ear to the brain

Visual processing: interpreting the visual world

Wernicke area: an area of the brain that is responsible for understanding and comprehending speech; located in the temporal lobe of the brain

Wildtype: gene with no mutation

Zonisamide (ZONEGRAN®): an anti-convulsant medication used to treat adult epilepsy

BIOGRAPHIES

JONATHAN FORBES, MD

Dr. Jonathan Forbes is a fellowship-trained, board-certified neurosurgeon with expertise and interest in open and minimally-invasive approaches for treatment of pathology of the cranial base. He has a long and distinguished history of academic recognition, commitment to excellence, and service to his country. Following the events of 9/11, Dr. Forbes enrolled in the Health Professions Scholarship Program with the United States 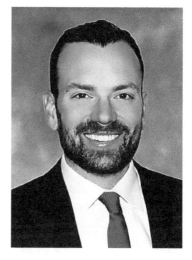 Air Force. While attending medical school at the University of Pittsburgh in Pittsburgh, Pennsylvania and completing his neurosurgical residency at Vanderbilt University in Nashville, Tennessee, he was the recipient of numerous national accolades. Following the completion of his chief year of neurosurgical residency at Vanderbilt in 2013, Dr. Forbes went on to fulfill a 4-year commitment with the U.S. Air Force that included a 6-month deployment to the Bagram Air Force Base in Afghanistan. After honorable discharge from the military, he completed a minimally-invasive skull base fellowship at Weill Cornell Medical Center in New York City under the guidance of Dr. Theodore Schwartz. Currently, Dr. Forbes is an assistant professor and program director for UC's Department of Neurosurgery. To date, Dr. Forbes has contributed to over 50 peer-reviewed publications.

ABDELKADER MAHAMMEDI, MD

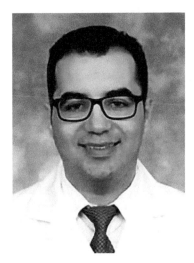

Dr. Abdelkader Mahammedi is an assistant professor of Neuroradiology at the University of Cincinnati Medical Center. He is a graduate of the University of Algiers medical school. He completed a postdoctoral research fellowship in Diagnostic Radiology at Johns Hopkins Hospital, Baltimore, MD, followed by residencies in both Nuclear Medicine and Diagnostic Radiology. Subsequently, Dr. Mahammedi went on to gain a Neuroradiology fellowship at the Cleveland Clinic Imaging Institute, Ohio. His specialty interests include brain tumors, stroke, head and neck imaging, and functional magnetic resonance imaging (fMRI). Dr. Mahammedi has contributed to over 20 peer-reviewed publications, including lead author of multiple articles in high-impact journals. He has recently published numerous multicenter and global COVID-19 related articles, which were featured in the international media; 200 newspapers, CNN, BBC, NPR, local televised broadcasts, and the 2020 RSNA Press Release. His work has been considered the first and largest study in the literature that systematically characterized neurological symptoms and neuroimaging features in hospitalized COVID-19 patients. Dr. Mahammedi has received numerous awards and honors, including being selected as a semi-finalist for the prestigious Cornelius Dyke Award of the American Society of Neuroradiology (ASNR) 2021, and the Best Case Award at the American Institute of Radiologic Pathology (AIRP) in Neuroradiology. He has also received a Top-Cited Article Award in 2014-2015 for his work in the Journal of Thoracic Imaging from the Society of Thoracic Imaging (STR) meeting, where he introduced a novel technique for early detection of pulmonary hypertension on CT scans.

SOMA SENGUPTA, MD, PHD, FRCP

Dr. Soma Sengupta is a neurologist who has trained at the University of Cambridge in England, Beth Israel Deaconess Medical Center, and Boston Children's Hospital in Boston, Massachusetts. She completed her neuro-oncology fellowship with training from Massachusetts General Hospital, Dana Farber Cancer Institute, and Brigham and Women's Hospital in Boston, Massachusetts. She is a board-certified neurologist and a neuro-oncologist. As a 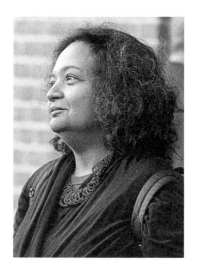 neuro-oncologist, Dr. Sengupta prescribes chemotherapy and takes care of the brain tumor survivorship needs of glioblastoma and other central nervous system cancer patients with her team. She attributes much of her inspiration to her patients and their journeys, including a childhood friend of hers who died from brain cancer. It has become extremely important for her to improve the survival outcomes and quality of life for this group of patients. In her free time, Dr. Sengupta enjoys spending time with her daughters, Amita and Maya. She is studying for a Master's in Business Administration with a focus in healthcare and completing an Integrative Medicine fellowship through the Andrew Weil Center for Integrative Medicine in Tuscon, Arizona, an opportunity made possible by the Schiff Scholarship Fund. Currently, Dr. Sengupta is the director of Medical Neuro-Oncology and Associate Director of the Brain Tumor Center at the University of Cincinnati and leads a multi-disciplinary team of clinicians and scientists. Dr. Sengupta has contributed to over 70 peer-reviewed publications and mentored many individuals over the years. She has inventions that are patented. In addition, Dr. Sengupta has been in the news and the radio shows for her diverse interests and research. In 2018, Dr. Sengupta published her children's book for brain tumor and cancer patients, entitled *Boo-boos and Butterflies*. Dr. Sengupta is the current holder of the Harold C. Schott Endowed Chair from the Department of Neurosurgery at the University of Cincinnati.

ACKNOWLEDGEMENTS

The authors would like to thank the patients and their families for their bravery and generosity in sharing their brain tumor journeys. Without them, this book would not be possible. The authors would also like to thank the following individuals for their contributions in creating this book:

- The Harold C. Schott Endowed Chair from the Department of Neurosurgery, the University of Cincinnati for protecting Soma Sengupta's time for research and educational endeavors.

- Mario Zuccarello, MD, Brett Kissela, MD, Joseph Cheng, MD, David Plas, PhD, and John Tew, MD, for their never-ending support.

- Val Cook, Sig Tumlin, Ashley Grizzle Soeder, and Bob Schultz for donating additional funds to make the book open access and for donating funds for the illustrations. They also contributed to proofreading the chapters about their respective loved ones.

- Ikumi Kayama, MA, for the detailed medical illustrations.

- Shivani Ghoshal, MD, for the front cover image.

- Brent Arehart for copyediting.

- Val Cook for donating a piece of Columbus Cook's artwork for the book.

- Daniel Pomeranz Krummel, PhD, and Alan Jobe, MD, PhD,
  for proofreading the book, as well as Ashley Grizzle Soeder,
  Val Porter Cook and Bob Schultz for proofreading their loved one's
  respective chapters.

- Hilary Perez, PhD, for her assistance with the Institutional Review
  Board review (2019-1403).